I0449056

# AFRICA SHOULD GET "THERE" TOO

*Alfani Sumaili Yoyo*

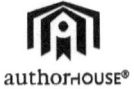

authorHOUSE®

*AuthorHouse™ UK Ltd.*
*500 Avebury Boulevard*
*Central Milton Keynes, MK9 2BE*
*www.authorhouse.co.uk*
*Phone: 08001974150*

*©2012. Alfani Sumaili Yoyo. All rights reserved*

*No part of this book may be reproduced, stored in a retrieval system, or transmitted by any means without the written permission of the author.*

*Published by AuthorHouse    10/22/2012*

*ISBN: 978-1-4567-4697-1 (sc)*
*ISBN: 978-1-4567-4696-4 (hc)*
*ISBN: 978-1-4567-4695-7 (e)*

*Library of Congress Control Number: 2011903005*

*Any people depicted in stock imagery provided by Thinkstock are models, and such images are being used for illustrative purposes only.*
*Certain stock imagery © Thinkstock.*

*This book is printed on acid-free paper.*

*Because of the dynamic nature of the Internet, any web addresses or links contained in this book may have changed since publication and may no longer be valid. The views expressed in this work are solely those of the author and do not necessarily reflect the views of the publisher, and the publisher hereby disclaims any responsibility for them.*

# CONTENTS

To my partner and best friend, Louise Ndolandola Mwemedi, who did not allow my weaknesses to snuff her love out but who concentrated on my strengths and accepted to cherish and complete me in every other aspect of life. Your love always motivated me to complete this book. I have chosen to love you unconditionally.

To my dear mama, Regina Byabula Nyassa, who often taught me leadership skills by example and unceasingly showed me how to become the responsible and caring man I am today. The type of love, kindness, esteem, and respect you showed to mankind is the sole spur of this book.

To all future leaders of Africa: You are the only hope left for this beautiful continent to come out of such a vexing deadlock. We believe you can if you would dare. Be leaders enough!

**S.Y. Alfani**

# Preface

This is a book written to people in transit, those taking a walk from a certain point of departure to a known yet unreachable destination. It's destined for an audience that understands it shouldn't remain motionless. It's all about development. Development, according to this version, is a walk from Here (where people are today) to There (where they long to be tomorrow). The word "unreachable" here sounds quite misleading, for it tends to mean that development cannot be achieved; it implies that all the nations we have dubbed "developed" should not be called so. Those nations should be referred thusly.

In my context, "unreachable" means that development is not something for which you can pat yourself on the back or exchange high-fives in a celebratory mood—as if to mean, "Yes, we have made it and now we shouldn't bother about anything else, so let's sit and enjoy." Rather, it's something that one pursues endlessly. It resembles some computer games in which a hundred points is the highest score but to which one qualifies from fifty points. Maybe all those developed countries today have already reached fifty or sixty but are still playing to get the highest score they can. Africa is too stagnant, perhaps below ten; it still has a lot to do to reach even fifty. In such a game, one hundred would be a kind of drive for the player to aim higher—to strive for the best.

So, development is well known to all but too demanding. However, that is exactly the risk Africa should take. Perhaps the African Union motto should be: "*The Quest for an Impossible Mission.*" This would be a powerful reminder.

I love Africa—not because I was born in one of its corners and therefore I'm compelled to love it after all—but because I believe so much in the continent's potential and capability. Africa should be the most blessed continent to attract the entire world this much. All other people's eyes are focused on Africa, especially those who are aware of what its land holds. Being a pan-Africanist (in some broad sense of the word), I always thought that the best and perhaps the only service I could render to my fellow

Africans is to address some issues that I believe have halted the continent's progress and, to some extent, suggest how they could be remedied.

I've chosen to embark on this particular field knowing that these issues are not being addressed accordingly. Many books written around this topic so far have dealt with them superficially. There seems to be a terrible fear among members of our communities vis-à-vis our leaders. And this is because of the intimidating "One-master-has-the-right-to-decide-for-all" attitude most African leaders have adopted. Silence, therefore, seems to be the best option for most of the population, especially those at the grassroots level. Unfortunately, silence will not get us any further. Looking at our present state, it is more risky to keep quiet than to stand and speak out. The need for Africa to move from stagnancy is urgent, and so is the need to remove all the stumbling blocks.

As I'm not in the position to offer a detailed account of everything, I would like to warn my readers in advance that my silence on some other issues that might be pertinent, vital, and crucial should not be mistaken for fear. Certainly, the omission of such issues has more to do with the mastery of the topic at hand. I believe honesty is, or should be, the wisdom of a writer. Every writer should concede his limitations on certain topics. And as mentioned somewhere else in this preface, one must learn his swimming skills in shallow waters—instead of deep waters—where he can easily manage to come out before he drowns. I'm simply writing this book as an amateur, not as an old hand, when tackling all the issues I've covered.

The book you're holding is directly addressed to young people, for they stand a one hundred percent chance to rule our countries in the near future. In it they'll be able to catch some hints on those hindrances and barriers to our continent's development. In some chapters I'm speaking with such a realistic tone that would make some of you think I'm being uncharitable to our present leaders. However, I believe exposing the wrongs of African leaders does not mean loving them less—it is, in fact, a sign and an affirmation of loving Africa more. Therefore, the motivation behind this book could best be summarized in the following five points:

#1: If I appear to sound a little more against some of our actual leaders, it's because I totally believe that our leaders could play a major role in everything that should be attempted to achieve progress. So, I suppose, if they allow things to be done, they will. The opposite is also true. And that's what we have been witnessing: our leaders are our own barriers to development. Most of our leaders have been deeply involved in what would not get us any further. If all the dictators in Africa could only dictate that every single cent should contribute to the development of their countries—instead of coercively getting people gather them wealth—it may go well with everything else. If they could involve everyone—I mean every citizen, including those in opposition rallies—into the development venture, everything else may run smoothly very soon.

I'm convinced that opposition parties emerge every now and then as a result of alarming rate of corruption tolerated by our governments, mismanagement in the public sector, and fallacious and empty promises made by the regime in power. This, sometimes, prompts me to think that maybe there'd be no opposition parties in a country where corruption is dealt with accordingly, where leaders in power learn to manage and use the public treasure wisely, promises made (especially during election campaigns) are kept and fulfilled, and marginalized and disadvantaged ordinary nationals—especially the elderly and vulnerable—are looked after. I believe that's what we mean whenever the wish of building a fair and just society overwhelms us and, fortunately, everyone longs for it.

Our leaders are well-positioned. They have that chance to make changes. If our desire is to see Africa changed one day, then our leaders should dare to stand as catalysts, motivators, instructors and facilitators. They should be ready to say willingly and boldly: "Let's move, we've been standing here for so long." It's because they are so reluctant to issue such an exhortation that I sound a bit negative on them but I'm really not. I'm simply trying to state some facts, so to speak.

#2: The actual leaders are not the direct target audience for this book. Meanwhile, my sincere gratitude goes to those who have managed to make their countries look like the Western world. There's no need to mention their names here. We all know who they are and they also know who they are. We know the state of each country around the continent, and most of us have already allocated them positions—from the first to the last—on our own rankings. These leaders are so brave and inspiring. I'm convinced they'd agree with me when I say Africa can also get where other continents are today if only everyone could truly love their countries. They set a very good example to the continent.

This book is partly a support for their achievement but more of an encouragement—a guide, a self-help or a motivation for prospective leaders. My aim for writing it is to help us avoid some mistakes that left us deadlocked; but in case it doesn't do, one is always free to pick up any other avenue that could get us There quickly. To the remaining group, in this book they may discover some mistakes that ensnared us and perpetuated our downfall. I've tried to suggest how some of these mistakes could be avoided, and that's what I refer to as essential keys to develop a crumbling continent.

#3: I regard myself as one of those who are already tired of being cheated. The political system in Africa has failed us dismally. Our political leaders have been treating us cheaply all along. They have been indeed downplaying us. It's time we get rid of this by any means possible. My fear, however, is that half of my argument in this book, if not all, might be considered as some kind of retaliation. In order to guard my readers against that, I'd like to insist that they should treat this book like something offered as a help or a guide—not like a compilation of some absolute "do's."

However, if some of us are still content with all that's happening in their countries, I don't think I can find something better to offer them. I know it's a big challenge to share the same path with contented cheats trying to persuade them to stop their corrupt ways. Their short-sightedness would certainly stand in their way. My argument can only make sense to those, like myself, who can't stand the whole scenario any longer but it would certainly mean less to the rest. My hope is that these cheats will one day get their vision back and abhor the whole corrupt system. That's my hope. There's certainly the right way to run state affairs. That's what I'm advocating, and that's what any other responsible citizen must long for and advocate.

On the other hand, although one might be satisfied with the status quo in his country, he should always try to avoid discouraging his fellows who still hope for some change. If societies will outlive individuals, then advocating for change—even to the point of death—is the right thing to do because it will surely benefit the society some day, if not immediately. Take Abraham Lincoln, for example. He didn't live to witness the final emancipation of black Americans from slavery. But the proclamation he made brought about freedom to the entire black American Community many decades after his assassination. The same applies to Dr. Martin Luther King Jr.:

He didn't live out his dream, but his conviction and consistency in the advocacy for civil rights in the U.S. brought about freedom to the people of his color, even after his death. Recently, we witnessed that his dream and advocacy for civil rights are still alive through Barack Obama's election. The desire to change our continent must now compel us to do whatever it takes (except the use of machine guns) to change our leaders and all ordinary people alike.

#4: I do not want to be associated with a non-progressive continent full of leaders who are always forcing us to believe that colonization is the cause of all our misery. I want to be part of a world where slave trade and colonization would remain part of my history but not the cause of my misery. Such a world where people can still rise beyond their decades of dark history and tough experiences—and prove that their IQs are in perfect condition—is what I long to be part of.

Who but a freak would accept to live in a country deprived of roads, electricity, and medicines—while at the same time the so-called leaders drive the most expensive cars and live in the most fanciful houses? Who would accept to always go hungry to bed in a country with the most fertile and arable land, in a country with the highest reserves of diamond and oil? Who would be content in a country whose quarter of land is covered by rivers and lakes and yet has no potable water? A country with the most powerful sources of energy yet has houses with no electricity all around its cities? Who would settle in a country full of minerals that fails to create jobs for its citizens? I can't imagine such a person.

If exploitation by colonizers is said to have impoverished us, what are we to say to our own leaders who do the same every day? Sadly, history tells us that some of our own people facilitated the trade of slaves right here on our continent. And our ancestors are said to have believed that people taken into slavery did not survive. Now, though, we know that some of them made it to the destination while many of them perished along the way. Those among us who facilitated to capture slaves must have been informed of these captives' fate: that they died in numbers on their way to some unknown place. But they did not care what would happen to their brothers so long as they get sugar, salt, and clothes from Caucasians. Yet everyone else around our world knows that's how pathetically selfish an African is even today.

To me, independence means telling whites "Go back to Europe. We shall continue this work ourselves." Unfortunately, the work referred to was none other than the extension of exploitation by a handful of our own people. We fought tooth and nail to get Europeans out of our countries under the pretext that they were exploiting us, but we put our hands on both cheeks watching our own people who are so wicked than even a hundred Hitlers. The truth is, exploitation by our own people is worse than that of colonizers, and it's so hurtful because it's not what we expect of them. We chased Europeans from our countries even after they had built us everything we see today in our nations, but we continue entertaining our own people even after destroying everything they did not build. What a catastrophe!

The desire of an African is the same that anyone else has elsewhere on our globe: We want to drive on good roads, we want food for everyone, we want to live in electrified houses, we want to drink potable water, we want to see proper medication and appropriate tools in our hospitals and clinics, we want to see our leaders being treated equally by the law in our courtrooms, and we want to get employed after graduation. Our governments must take the lead. That's our heartbeat and yet another motivation for this book.

#5: And, finally, as I said earlier, I've written this book as an amateur—not as a political analyst, a land manager, a clergyman, a HIV/AIDS eradication specialist, or anything else. Of course a specialist in one of these fields would definitely have some different views. Therefore, if you're a specialist in one of the fields I've touched in this book, don't feel disappointed when you find that I've given some details that you think are unnecessary or fail to hit the proper target. And don't blame me for rather going beyond the boundaries of the topic. Remember here the difference is: you're a specialist and I'm not. This is the type of help or guide I can ever get to offer when interfering with your specialty.

I'm caught in between, so to speak. I'm afraid to get into deep waters that may make it difficult for me to offer what I would like to maintain as help. All I sincerely would like to offer is help, and one can give it in accordance with his competence. This is what I'm capable of doing. In my view, you're reading nothing more or nothing less than what I'm really able to offer. I've emptied myself, so to speak. Try to ask me for more and you'd soon label me as the confused man of the century; likewise ask me for less and you'd soon discover the level of my hypocrisy. Therefore, I ask my readers to be content with the little or the more, or whatever they please to call it, I've offered in this book. Those five points are the basis of this book.

However, I acknowledge having omitted or rather presented very briefly some other important issues. As you'd notice, the land issue alone is covered in three chapters in this book. I have one clear reason for doing this. My emphasis on land is intentional. The impression that one may get from the land's coverage in this book is that I give it more value. Such an impression is true; and I also have to admit that this is quite personal for several reasons.

I've never felt proud to be a citizen of such a fertile and rich country like the Democratic Republic of Congo (DRC) that marked its independence in 1960 (a decade and a half before I was born), that still imports fresh tomatoes from a distant country like South Africa even after three decades of my existence. That's more than corruption. I don't think our world would find any right word to describe that.

Furthermore, I'm always disturbed whenever I try to think on behalf of some young Ethiopians who might be doing a course that teaches students that their land doesn't have the right ingredients to grow some food plants but that is not the case with other countries on the continent. My worry is what could be the reaction of these youth when they learn that their country shares its borders with some fertile lands? What if they learn that there are countries like the DRC that do not even need fertilizers to boost their lands? When they discover this, I believe their first question would be: "If that's true, why should we starve to death or expect some food supply from other parts of the world?" And, guess their reaction; I believe it would sound something closer to this: "They hate us or else there should also be some hell going on there!" It's the latter that fits to describe it: there's indeed more than hell going on in those countries like DRC.

Besides, who can allow his mind to concede that a country with arable land would depend on the World Food Programme (WFP) to feed its population? And, who would expect WFP supply in a country that didn't encounter any flood, drought, hurricane or tsunami? Yet some of our nations are in such an embarrassing situation. They can't do without WFP.

In my own view and that of many others, our land alone has the potential to eradicate hunger on the entire continent without resorting to handouts from outside. There should be neither beggars of food by the streets of African cities or villages nor kids dying somewhere for lack of a cassava, a potato, or an apple at least, to quench their hunger. At this time of the world's history there shouldn't be any country toiling to cover some food debts or begging other countries to write off their food debts—that's an embarrassment beyond description!

I used to believe that our continent had some values that would make her proud to be free from getting any debt as ridiculous as food debt. I used to think that Africa could proudly put some mechanism in place for preventing any such humiliation from happening and so defend the dignity and the pride of the African man that we always profess.

Unfortunately, the day-to-day experience shows the opposite. It seems that we don't care much about our dignity when an issue takes a national stance. Perhaps at a certain level all these stories become mere village chats. And, if really, the dignity and pride of an African are limited to the affairs of a village and not extending to the national level, then our mutation—or what some of us would refer to as civilization or advancement—is more to our own shame. It's utterly sordid to see Africans being strangled in public and announced over the world's leading media networks for not having paid some food's debts while sitting on the most fertile land of the planet. Shame on us!

These are some of the reasons why land is the most discussed subject in this book; but any other issues currently affecting our development are equally important. Some of these issues were well highlighted by President Barack Obama in his remarks to the Ghanaian Parliament in July 2009. It was his first trip to sub-Saharan Africa, and he spoke out his heart on Africa's destitution. Now for me this was a great coincidence. My book was about to undergo the final full edit before getting into the marketing phase when Obama delivered his moving speech in Accra. I had to notify my agent that the number of words of my script had raised; and I was ready to add a few dollars on the initial full edit quotation for the words that were accrued from quotes from president Obama's address. You will come across some of those quotes later. I'm proud to share the same ideas with the American president.

Finally, I don't want to leave my readers clueless on the fact that I've used a lot of colloquialism throughout this book. This is partly because of my target audience (the youth) but mainly because I rather wanted to keep it simple, more like a one-on-one conversation or like a talk show in broadcast media.

# Introduction

It all started as a wish—a wish that everyone could take the following words as his personal creed, mean every single word his lips utter, and proclaim it everywhere:

*I love Africa. I will live in Africa for the rest of my days. I will be buried in Africa. Africa is in my heart when I wake up, when I talk, when I eat, and when I sleep. I'm tired of seeing my continent on the last row, but I'm determined to do whatever I can to get it to the front row.*

Our continent is a beautiful place where you find all kinds of people, riches, resources, and different weather just as you find them on other continents. Its soil is fertile, though some places are dry. Its people are hard-working. They're hospitable and caring, loving and kind, acceptable and charitable, sharing and friendly just like others. Natural, beautiful fauna and flora replenish various corners of the continent. Parks and games are still as beautiful and attractive as they were made.

Rivers, lakes, dams, and oceans cover the continent all around. The sun shines just as usual, the rain falls abundantly, the moon is clearly seen by night, the wind blows to and fro, and the fresh air is still natural. Everything natural and artificial on other continents is still found wrapped in the magnificent African nature alone. But an important number of its population is deserting it every year in search for green pastures. Their complaint is always the same: Africa does not offer them facilities they wish to have. It's all summarized in one sentence: "Africa is not developed." Development is at issue here.

While African countries fail to retain the big number of their population leaving every year, Europe and America are, on the other side, complaining about those illegally landing on their soil on a daily basis. For many young men in Africa, the pasture seems to be greener outside. According to them, beautiful cities, clean stuff, healthy and abundant food, modern education facilities, and especially job opportunities are the main driving forces behind their illegal migration.

In order to stop this massive illegal migration, it seems that the solution is to develop our countries. We must develop them not only to avoid brain drain or to keep Africans in Africa but for us to live like everybody else in the West, for example; and meet the standard of this century.

I believe migration is not bad when it's about exploring other parts of the world so as to mingle and know other people's cultures. But when it becomes a massive, one-way migration, it turns out to be a dangerous hindrance to any country's development.

Now, even at this moment, I'm so afraid that everyone might leave his dirty and careless country in search for green pastures outside. I feel I can even encourage them to do so if they're searching for jobs when their countries can't offer them. Perhaps that could make their leaders come back to their senses and, at least, do something for the rest of the population (mainly women and children) remaining in their countries as a strategy to persuade them to stay behind. This could be a nice strategy to get supporters for their subsequent unending terms and also have subjects to rule over. Yet, on the other hand, I'm afraid that they (leaders) might get more careless to a handful of women and children who remain behind.

Encouraging this illegal migration could be the oddest thing one would do. Stop it? Only a fool can keep someone where all future prospects are shattered and hopelessness prevails. But despite whatever that could breed ultimately, I believe one must stop these fellows from deserting their countries so to get them rally behind what could be called "conscientization march" against our leaders. As was emphasized by President Barack Obama in Ghana, African youth have the power to hold their leaders accountable and to build institutions that serve the people. They can conquer disease, end conflicts, and make change from the bottom up. That should be the aim of our "conscientization march."

We possess all the resources capable to change our continent into something like (or more than) Europe or America. In order to attain such change, we need to get our leaders to unlearn all the selfish ambitions and "what's-good-for-me-is-good-enough" attitude they've been practicing for years. This would help them refocus and learn to sympathize with everyone else in their countries, especially the downtrodden peasants on the grassroots level.

Besides, I don't see how deserting your country would miraculously translate into change. Running away might only stimulate greedy leaders to continue mismanaging public resources. And that's what we've been witnessing on our continent so far. One strategy that could bring about change in our countries is to keep addressing the problem, as I'm doing now; complaining and shouting to our leaders with one voice and uncompromisingly, on a face-to-face encounter. I'm sure some of us would accuse such practice of demeaning any reverence we owe our "kings" in Africa. But I'm of the view that any careless king is not king enough to be revered. So our presence on this continent, and especially in our countries, would somehow be a bugbear to them and it can make them stop—or at least relent or even reverse. That could be the beginning of our breakthrough.

Sadly, we're always afraid to face our leaders for fear of risking abductions or something even worse. Though this is true, I haven't, on the other hand, learnt or heard of any revolution that was achieved by a bunch of cowards. All great moments in history were marked by great sacrifices. All revolutionaries and pioneers in the world's history were always brave and ready to be martyred for the cause. And revolution always takes time. After all, it's none of my wishes that blood should be shed to get our leaders to understand our bottom line.

Every one of us longs for development, and we all need it to materialize. It is no wonder why we are so attracted to countries that have modern facilities and accessible infrastructure. How can we attain it, then? That's what we must seek endlessly. Development is something of public interest. Each one of us longs to see it materialize. It shouldn't be like some mythical word in a fictitious world or in a novel or a fairy tale. Development is a real word, one that no other word in the dictionary can ever define correctly: It means buildings, roads, modern facilities, technology and infrastructures in a given country.

Above all, I also think that knowing the types of agents or systems we keep on encountering throughout our history is important in helping us to easily know who might quickly support our endeavor for development and those who wouldn't. From the independence era to date, I've noticed four types of systems that have ever existed in Africa. There might be more but the following are those I've noticed so far:

**1.** *Those who said: "Push it, let's get going."* This category is largely made of those who got some leadership positions straight from Europeans as result of independence in mid-twentieth century. They keenly claimed their land back or, as we say, "struggled for the liberation of our countries from foreign occupation." Or rather, as echoed in some freedom songs, "They got up and stood for their rights without giving up the fight." Well, anybody can do that when he feels oppressed or deprived of his rights.

The process was all good and worth it, I guess. But I think it ignored some good procedures. In order to explain this correctly I will make use of another tradition which I think is quite similar. During my early years of primary education in my country, the Democratic Republic of Congo, then Zaïre; we often had intern teachers from colleges. In order for them to perform well, they were always confined to working (for one or two weeks) under the supervision of our regular teachers. And they could only be allowed to carry out the task by themselves after that period. I know this is practiced in other countries.

My partner and best friend Louise Mwemedi is a medical doctor. She also told me they're first submitted to the tutelage of a qualified and experienced medical doctor before they can be allowed to perform any surgical operation alone. And I know that so many fields, especially technical ones, apply this. This process is very important for the intern or the trainee to learn to convert a number of theories learnt into practice or even sometimes to acquire new knowledge. This helps him to apply his long observations to the real world. Practice is different from theory in some way, and this is a matter of experience. This period of apprenticeship may seem insufficient or even sometimes meaningless, but it is the only time that the trainee gets in touch with his career. He learns some concrete and necessary skills—in a routine way under supervision—that would help him for the rest of his life. This is perhaps an unsuitable illustration but it can give us some hints on how we were supposed to do. Unfortunately, as remarked earlier, that is what was ignored.

After our countries became independent, we started forcing Europeans to step out. We forgot these Westerners managed our countries for many years and knew a lot more about our countries than we did at that time. Perhaps the ousting of Europeans was because of anger, or that we simply wanted to retaliate. However, to blame someone for this act may also be arrogant. Oppression in itself is bad and wrong, but oppression in your own yard and for your own property is unbearably worse. But if we want to be wise, shouldn't we start by trying to control the world within us, at least, if we can't control the outside one? Maybe it was too early for people to yield to all those complicated psychological principles and formulas, or perhaps it was completely unbearable. I know I can't invent any suitable formula for this. I would be a hypocrite if I professed to do well under such a fierce fire. Maybe I would also do preciously little in the face of that predicament. In other words, I shouldn't issue orders to those in the battlefield while I'm exempted from it—safe and at ease.

Frankly, I never cease to ask myself what I could have done if I happened to live under colonization or apartheid. Plainly, I'm not sure what I could have done if I were Nelson Mandela, for instance. Nevertheless, I think what matters here is not what a resentful individual like me could do, but rather what the humanity as a whole ought to do when their world is at stake. That's what inspired Mandela, and it's perhaps what could have guided me, too.

Though I can't suggest any right solution to the problem, I know, on the other hand, that revenge doesn't delight in letting another person off. Revenge enjoys a draw game and it is indeed a draw game propaganda. Those of us who love soccer know that from a draw comes extra time and then sometimes a penalty shootout. The only thing I hate in soccer is a draw in a quarterfinal, a semi-final, or the final. I'd rather like to see a team win or lose the game in the allocated time. It's only then that I could be spared from heartache. A draw tends to perpetuate the game and drags with it other things that are too hard to bear sometimes: heartache, waste of time, lack of concentration, and other funny feelings. Resentment is not good in any case. Often the tiring and stressful game to both players and spectators is the one that goes on and on for a long time; and so is a resentful attitude. I know this illustration cannot succeed in giving an accurate picture of the whole scenario. However, I used it to show how retaliating and resentful our spirits were and still are animated.

Sometimes it is good to let the opposing party off, pass or proceed. I guess you'd notice how dodgy I am in using the words "win" and "lose." These words carry with them the wrong connotation, and they're often misleading and provocative whenever used to refer to confrontations between human beings. Naturally—and I guess we've all noticed it—people have an inborn longing for winning rather than losing. Nobody would accept to be referred to as a loser; that's almost an insult to most of us. That's why I think the expression "letting the opposite party off, go, proceed, or pass" can work perfectly in matters involving human beings instead of the terms "win" and "lose".

"Push it, let's get going" sounds more like an old car that fails to start by itself unless it gets a push. And, unfortunately, that's how most of our countries were ruled after independence. It was more like guesswork being performed. Just like one guy in a movie who was asked by his friends to explain what he was trying to do to get them out of trouble when they were stuck and who suddenly answered: "How should I know? I'm just trying to guess!" I believe if we invite a few of those leaders to a panel discussion today and ask them to tell us how they were doing their things, some would honestly say that a great deal of what they did was just being guessed at. Sadly enough, even today, after almost half a century removed from colonization, most of our countries are still ruled under this principle.

When pushing something, you're likely to get tired and react out of anger or stress. If the thing that is being pushed works after a push, there's some kind of relief. But if it doesn't, even after a long attempt, some people surrender, some throw the item away, others sacrifice it or tear it down at once or give more attention only to the part that is still working. That's why we can still notice the same syndrome in Africa even today: Some sectors are forgotten, surrendered, sacrificed or even neglected completely. Because we have a lot of minerals and they make the country money, our government treats this sector as one of the few parts of the machine that is working without complications, so it should be given more attention. And because we failed to maintain our tractors, even after many attempts to get them work, the agricultural sector seems to us the most complicated and so it should be neglected. That's when hunger comes in and as a result, everybody else, especially those in the cabinet, spends their time in inventing some shrewd formulas to get diamond or gold in some illegal ways.

The "trial and error" regimes got us all the trouble we have to bear now. Most of those countries that decided to keep the so-called "oppressors" within their borders even after such "unbearable experiences" and "hardships" are performing much better today compared to those that felt it was "totally unbearable" to cohabit with "enemies". I'm convinced those countries understood that Westerners were like the schoolteachers or those experienced medical doctors or supervisors I mentioned earlier, and so they considered themselves as trainees or interns who needed some clear instructions for a better performance which they unquestionably acquired. Those countries that ignored this process are still struggling even after several decades of independence. And, unfortunately, the blame is still put on "imperialists" up to now. What a tragedy!

And here is the irony: Even today I feel like we still need to get Westerners back in all our countries to put an end to "push it, let's get going" because it didn't—and probably won't—get us any further. Perhaps they know some good strategies essential for the management of our countries that we have never figured out or won't probably discover now. But that's yet another wish. And anyway, how can't they know the secret of our countries after having managed them for many years? I would like to make something clear here. To invite Caucasians back has nothing to do with cowardice, as some of us were brought to believe; rather, it's acknowledging our own limitations and that is wisdom. And (this is true in any way and it gives much hope to any trainee) there's no guarantee that the supervisor or the instructor will remain knowledgeable than his trainee all the time. The only advantage the supervisor or the instructor has at a particular time is that of knowing his subject or specialty before the trainee. But the trainee can sometimes become more knowledgeable than his supervisor. It all depends on the trainee's attitude toward his supervisor, his willingness, and the effort he employs to learn.

In other words, allowing some Westerners to work as trainers and supervisors is true reconciliation in an unhidden manner. I don't want to put this in some diplomatic words because one reason why I hate diplomatic speeches is that the speakers seem to be using words (not carefully, as they would say, but cunningly) that they alone know the meaning. It's easy for the speaker to deny what he said a few minutes ago if he used a diplomatic language. They're so evasive. They can easily convince the audience that they misunderstood them when they're about to catch them on the words they had just uttered. What I mean is that we should forgive any wrong that happened between Westerners and us and should allow them to live with us without holding any grudges.

On this issue, it's not easy to diverge from the majority without appearing like something worse than a rebel or a lunatic. But we must allow Westerners to settle in our countries in numbers. That could be a successful surgeon to "push it, let's get going" in most of our states. Once they settle, we must view them as "facilitators" who are only passing on their knowledge to trustworthy and smart chaps who would do the same some other time in the near future. The whole circle of knowledge sharing should only produce facilitators in the end. That's where our development lies: a knowledge economy.

There's another vice to this. Our tendency to keep a distance between Westerners and us is not because they come from other continents or have a different skin color but often it's because we think they're extremely smart that if you allow them to take an inch they may end up taking a mile. I'm not sure about this, at least for the moment, but I'm sure I'm not trying to be evasive. I've learned that intelligent people are also the most helpful and sharing—this is a matter of experience. They know that, given all the time and resources of the world, they could never turn them into anything useful unless they team up. They're aware that all hangs on interdependency. Any smart person knows that he can never have enough time to sit and think about formulas to invent and maintain machinery—and be at the same time the mechanic to fix a screw that breaks loose— invent an aircraft and be the pilot at the same time. They believe in teamwork and know that knowledge sharing is the key to productivity. They may start the fist step; perhaps the second or third, but won't surely continue the rest of the way. It's only businessmen who tend to be reluctant to share their ideas sometimes. Therefore, intelligent and learned people or scholars are the loveliest people to live with. While businessmen would like to draw all the money to themselves; learned people wouldn't like to pilot all the aircrafts they invent even when they are tempted to, so to speak.

At least this is one of my formulas to bring "push it, let's get going" to an end. If you have any other better formula, implement it. All we must diligently seek to avoid is guesswork, and here, as I said earlier, learning to acknowledge one's limitations is the first step.

**2. Those who say:** *"Ngai nde nakobongisa yango?"* This is a Lingala statement meaning, "Is it my responsibility to fix it?" Lingala is one of the national languages in both the DRC and neighboring Republic of Congo, also known as Congo-Brazzaville.

I've noticed that leaders who utter such statements are among those who assumed some leadership positions mostly through violence—usually not democratically elected—and never endeavour to improve anything. They put the blame on those who ruled before them. Their attitude is, "Nothing should be expected from us to make things work." Their conviction is that a lot of stuff went wrong already and they should be left so. And if anything should be improved at all, then that's not their responsibility. They'd say or think: "I'm not here to mend what I didn't twist; So many things are broken, there's no need to bother about their reparation; They've started destroying the wall, let's help them take it down; It's all their fault, we can't help;" or "The tree is curved, is it our responsibility to straighten it up?"

Despondently, these leaders don't think in terms of whether it's possible or impossible for the matter to get fixed, they'd rather think that it's not worth trying. They deliberately ignore that in every case there's always chance for spoiled stuff to get repaired, for broken walls to be rebuilt, and for bending trees to be straightened up again, at any rate when they're still young. What such leaders would never do is trying to take the trouble of repairing twisted stuff, rebuilding broken walls or straightening up bending trees. They don't try this because—and I fully believe this—they know that some things can easily function when given enough attention. So they better ignore them, perhaps in order to avenge their predecessors who caused the damage.

If what prompts them to be so careless is revenge, it means they refuse to "pay for the pot they did not break." The game must end in a draw (one-all). But on the other hand, to their successors, this would give them low marks on the "evaluation scale" they leave behind. Any leader who fails to leave a legacy behind, especially after several decades in the office, is probably putting up a big poster with the following inscription in bold: "My failure exposes my brain." You are a nobody if you can't fill up the "achievement column" of your autobiography.

Here is the bottom line for the rest of us: it's our task as leaders to straighten things up, to rebuild broken walls and to mend everything that was spoiled. We are the right people for that task. We must forget about the past as soon as we climb the ladder of leadership. After more than forty years from independence we have no reason to blame anybody for our underdevelopment. And it is a blatant waste of time to keep on blaming someone for the past mistakes. The past is the only part of our lives we can never fix. It remains unchangeable. So there's no reason to sit down with our victim attitude. The only parts of our lives we can change, if we so wish, are the present and the future. We have it all in our hands. And so we must live this present moment preparing for the future. We shouldn't waste any other time trying to think over the mess of the past. Africa is not the only continent that was colonized, and we are not the only race that was ill-treated. Our friends on other continents seem to have been moving to the pace of the world despite their awful past than we are. We have been holding on the past though we know we can't change it. And the most horrible thing is that we have never been ashamed of our most disgusting attitude: that Westerners "owe us." They owe us nothing. What they took is nothing compared to what we have left, and yet we are the most unproductive race and underdeveloped people on the face of the earth. What a shame!

Let's face this: The best you can draw out of the past is any potential lesson you could learn for the future. But if you can't learn any, then leave the past alone. It means you have nothing to do with it. It's time to concentrate on the future now. If you ask me why, I should answer you that it's because when you become a leader, nothing is about yourself. And if you're living now, everything is about the future: the houses you build, the children you beget, the friends you make, and even your behaviour are all bearing future implications. They're all accountable in the future, especially when you're gone. If someone failed before you, it doesn't mean you should purposely fail, too. His failure should pave the way for your success. If he did nothing good, you should do everything good. How pleasant it is to achieve a great success right after a great failure! There's an overwhelming joy in that. Consider the following statement as a personal motivation: "Be ready to attempt to put the right side up when things are upside down."

**3. Those who say: *"If I only had good advisers!"*** These leaders are eager to achieve great things when they assume some higher positions but they blame their entourage. They feel their failure has something to do with their association with a wrong mob: their entourage make them deviate. Always they hear things like: "Now is your turn, don't ever mess it up;" "If you won't make money now, forget about getting wealthy in your entire life;" "Opportunities such as these don't come twice;" or "You have killed an elephant."

These leaders would like to achieve a number of projects, but they're strayed before they get to the implementation phase. Trouble arises around them as soon as they start preparing for action. Nothing gets done properly, especially when they delegate. Everybody tends to gather as much as he can. They need everything but development.

Leaders in this category try by all means to resist this problem but (and this is shocking), they don't seem to be fighting it fervently. Because of their indifference, they gradually get dragged to the corrupt side. In most cases, such leaders fail to influence their entourage. The odd thing about this scenario is that the game seems to be opposing one man against the mob, and in such a game the score can always be predicted. Finally, they end up giving up some of their noble dreams for greed and self-enrichment.

And there's always something peculiar about their entourage. Often people in their entourage had either served some former corrupt regimes and have become experts in mismanagement or else they're greatly inspired by the second group's attitude: "Those who were here before did nothing but piling up possessions." They're eventually drawn into the second group and they're quickly persuaded that they shouldn't take much trouble doing a job that seems nobody's business. Who cares, anyway? So they finally indulge into squandering public resources.

Another odd thing about this mob is that most of them are related to these leaders in one way or another: They're either from these leaders' tribes or regions. Here's when tribalism starts taking root. They persuade their "relatives" (leaders) to ignore any plan that would benefit everybody else—in this case, it means other tribes. Sacrificing the country's budget on the expense of other people and places for the benefit of a small ethnic or tribal group becomes the order of each day in such regimes. Projects aimed at improving everybody's life countrywide are easily stifled. They rather prefer to maintain the gap between the haves and have-nots. I mean they believe there should be a sharp difference between the tribe that is leading the country and other tribes. State affairs become completely a tribal issue. Consequently, other tribes are regarded as foreigners or parasites, more like intruders who are only taking chance. Worse still is their attitude to constantly compare themselves with other tribes that ruled the country before—the comparison is based on how those other tribes enriched themselves from the country's resources without involving others. So I can say that their administration is motivated by revenge and the pursuit of wealth. It's a big shame to join such a competition. It's a game that benefits no one in the long run. Yet we have never realized that.

Why shouldn't we be proud of achieving what others failed to? Suppose tribe A did nothing for tribes B, C, or D; why should tribe B fall into the same trap? I believe when our minds are fully functioning and quite away from any type of such invented competition and futile revenge, tribe B would be compelled to do better than tribe A to gain people's praise and confidence and even beat the world's record at rising to the top against all the odds. It's amazing to see how we always drag tribalism in the government's affairs, no matter how disappointing it has been to many of our countries. Mature people would be pleased with nothing else but achieving something that was never done before. Some of us are relentlessly looking for such opportunities to unfold in our favour while others are simply messing them up. What a contrast!

When you're in pursuit of approval, popularity and fame, the "mess up and I'll show you how messy I am" principle can never work. The principle that could work is, "If you mess up I'll show you how tidy and organized I am." And only the latter could draw more people closer. Sadly, those who apply the first principle either intentionally or unintentionally ignore one fact: They hardly think they would step down some day (no matter after how many decades) and certainly another tribe would take the lead. I'm not sure what tribe A would think when tribe B gets the power, and likewise I don't know what tribe B would expect from tribe C when it climbs to the highest position and applies the same crooked and corrupt principle. Well, I'm not sure, but we've witnessed some of those former leaders complaining as if they knew nothing of that kind. From this experience, one can foresee how squeezed we shall be if we drag our tribes into government's affairs.

Any leader with good dreams must dare to stand alone against the corrupt mob. He must implement his projects and get rid of any corrupt adviser around him. Advisers can't always offer good advice because—even in a better world—none of them would be perfect. And we must always remember that an advice is only there for the taking; it's up to us to decide what to do with it. Advice is never a policy to be implemented; rather, it's an offer to be either taken or left alone, especially when it's tainted with corruption. Remember, if you buy into any corrupt advice, you'd ultimately suffer the consequence. In this case, our self-help statement could be: "If tribe A fails, tribe B must clean the mess and tidy up the place; then tribe C and others must do better than A and B.

**4. Those who say:** ***"Only development matters."*** Such leaders are only concerned about upgrading their countries. Their minds are so overwhelmed by one thing, and that is to upgrade their countries. They willingly forget about themselves to promote everybody. They're consumed with the desire to see everybody else climbing the ladder of success together with them. That's the right type of leadership! Our continent needs such leaders who have gone beyond individualism, people who have stopped focusing on themselves. I believe they should ask themselves: "What can man really gain during his brief time on earth if he illicitly gets everything he wants on the expense of others?" I know they also suggest an answer to their question: "Well, fame and praise and some kind of respect may temporarily be gained in the process, but shame would permanently stick to one's name afterward." Such people know that true fame, praise, and respect are gained not by climbing the ladder of success alone but by helping others climb it, too.

Many times people who aim at fame, praise, popularity, and respect find themselves in a complete confusion. That has proven to be a wrong starting point. Many people who started by focusing on themselves got disappointed and discouraged in the end. That's where you find all the tyrants of our continent listed: dictators such as Idi Amin of Uganda, Mobutu Sese Seko of Zaire (now DRC), Eyadema of Togo, and many others. But most of those who started with others and almost forgetting about fame, praise and all the likes were the most popular and respected men in the end.

So, start with yourself, with your heart full of the thrills of popularity and respect, you'd probably get nothing in the end. But start with others, with no idea of respect, fame and praise; start with the thrills of meeting other people's needs first, you'd surely become the most popular and respected man, even in the world ranking. That's why those men and women who forgot about themselves and had their hearts sold out for others rose above the rest: Nelson Mandela, Dr. Martin Luther King Jr., Mother Teresa, Mahatma Gandhi, and other people who could be referred to as "great souls" found themselves popular without even thinking of it.

Those who think this world is a "Wealth Exhibition Center," where everyone is expected to flaunt their wealth before they die, are completely mistaken. Even if it could be an exhibition center, African leaders should always know that nobody in their countries would take part in that event to admire their savings or their mansions. If that exhibition could happen at all, many would go there not to appreciate how smart their leaders are but they'd attend it with great expectation to get some leftovers—some kinds of shares. If they receive something, they would then applaud their leaders with much respect; and that would guarantee the fame and popularity of these leaders. But if they don't find what they're in for, they may still applaud in some fake manner. Perhaps it's because they're scared of their leaders' swords, and in that case they have no option than to do something to please their leaders—to applaud. And this is, unfortunately, the case in Africa. People applaud for things they'd rather not praise. They exhibit dances, and attend political rallies out of fear. They do things they'd rather not do at all simply to preserve their lives. But it's time we bring this to an end.

They may also applaud in a cheating way, just to get their leaders' approval at that particular event. And all that really breeds is a lifelong shame. Our self-help statement in this case would be: "Be a leader whose heart is on others—not yourself. Let 'Only development matters' be your slogan."

In conclusion, I personally appreciate those of our leaders who fall under the last category because they really defend the image of our continent. If Africa gets some credit at all, it's because of those countries. They wipe off some prejudices those outsiders, especially Westerners, are primarily filled with before they visit Africa. These countries manage to maintain some of their infrastructure like the West. One of the things that amaze me is that their schools and universities enroll students from other continents. These students do not simply register because they want to study somewhere in Africa but because they do not notice much difference between their schools back home and these ones in Africa. Now—and this is a terrifying truth—finding Western or Eastern students enrolled in schools or any institution of higher learning in some other parts of Africa is a dream that is impossible to be fulfilled because some of our schools aren't even worth bearing that name. They don't deserve to be called schools, colleges or universities at all. And if they're to be called so then those in the West should get a new name. One or the other should change its appellation.

That's a very good example to set! I wish everyone could be so highly motivated. I feel it's difficult but I know it's not impossible. Above all, I know that everyone of us wishes to see Africa developed, let's achieve it then! That's our only challenge.

# Chapter One

# Development: The African Dream?

I once read about someone who got lost in the mountains. In order to get out of them, he sought assistance from the campsite and was told: "You can't get there from here. You must start from the other side of the mountains." In the same way, no matter how much we long for development, it can't materialize unless we remember the height from which we missed the target and start afresh.

The word "development" is mentioned on a daily basis in every nation around the globe. In those nations already developed, I guess this word means to keep on progressing. But to developing nations, it would mean something else. For them it would mean to engage into a serious walk from "Here" to "There." It is realizing that they've spent too much time in one place and under the same conditions. So development to them would mean to make their environment look different—look better. It means they're not willing to keep the status quo any longer. It is to cross over to the other edge of the river and continue with the journey. It is being fed up with the same stuff. Development then seems to be nothing else but a journey from "Here" (where people are today) to "There" (where they long or dream to be tomorrow)—it is more than a change for better. It is a total change in all aspects of life. It is true that people feel development before they even need it. Before someone in Africa needs to live like an American for example, he first feels it. He feels he should live like an American.

He's overwhelmed by feelings of self-assurance that he is able to quit, to change everything, and live his best life now. This feeling prompts him to think he can live differently, he can enlarge, he can expand, he can transform, he's able to climb higher, and he can excel. However, we must also keep in mind that while every change is not improvement, every improvement is change. For example, you can change your office outlook by repositioning your tables and shifting your cupboards or shelves, but you can improve it by bringing in new furniture.

Even in my village, people feel the same. I'm not sure about other places, but I'm inclined to believe that none of us would sit and be content in a place where there's no potable water, electrified houses, good road infrastructure, health centers, and communication facilities. People always aspire for these things and they never stop dreaming big, no matter how poor their hamlet may look like.

Most of us dream to see skyscrapers around us. Not only to see them, but also to stay, work and live in them. We're dreaming to see our townships flourishing according to our needs. To accompany our kids to those most beautiful garden parks and playgrounds that make one wish he was a child again. To travel a thousand kilometers in few hours. To see clean and attractive public arenas. To see our food stores always full of healthier, tastier, and more delicious foods. To get employed whenever we need employment. We're dreaming to live the reality of magazines and movies— to live the Hollywood life, so to speak.

This means to get rewarded from our taxes (in those countries where taxes are paid) and also to enjoy our land's resources. And this is why I've just said we would like to enjoy our taxes and our natural resources: In some African countries people are now getting tired of paying taxes because it turns out to be a waste because nothing is gained from paying them. Yet in other countries the word tax seems to be either missing or deliberately skipped from their vocabulary.

I know what I'm talking about: it's not a parrot-fashion statement. Some citizens of those countries don't even know what the word "tax" implies. Maybe that is a shrewd way of squeezing them into a trap that would leave them without any right to criticize the government. Maybe! Yes, where would one get the guts to blame the government for not building a bridge or a road if he contributes nothing to the nation from all his income?

I also said that we would like to enjoy our natural resources. Some of our countries are so overwhelmingly blessed with them to the extent of making one think that the distributor was dozing when all these resources slipped out of his hands, dropping them in one place. Yet there's no slightest evidence showing they have them at all. They look no different from hell.

I mentioned earlier that people would like to see real things—tangible stuff—in their countries. They want to see their countries rebuilt, covered with all kinds of modern buildings (tall, short, small, big: painted in a mixture of colors) everywhere. They want to see investors at every corner—investors that are able to fill up their stores with goods responding to their demand. Africans never stop dreaming to attend universities like Melbourne, Paris, Cambridge, Oral Roberts, Harvard, and Oxford—right here in Africa. Their hope is to have those royal gardens and noble playgrounds from Melbourne, New York, Washington, Sydney, Paris, Stockholm, Ottawa, Nassau, London, California, Moscow, Cologne, Tokyo, Hong Kong, and Beijing—right here in Africa. They want to see their roads in good conditions: to have their breakfast in Cape Town, South Africa, and their supper in Cairo, Egypt. They want to see clean and spotless stuff around them. To get food—not just something edible, but food that is treated and stored in healthy conditions. If there is any place referred to as "paradise," then that is exactly our dream—to make Africa our heaven on earth.

Now here is where all the matter lies: How shall we get "There" from "Here?" We've got to move, after all! All other continents are already ahead of us. To put this in a simple way: How shall we get a paradise out of Africa? Also to mean how shall we get a paradise from a "fallen world?" In other terms, how shall our developing countries get developed? More plainly, how shall Malawi turn into Japan? (Let me clarify something here before I move on. To take Malawi in this illustration as the poorest country on the continent is as wrong as considering Japan to be the most developed country in the world. It's a simple comparison based on the difference between those two countries as far as development is concerned. Just take it like the DRC and the USA). Then, asking how Malawi shall turn into Japan is simply another way of asking how Africa shall turn into North America.

In our minds, we feel America though living in Africa. No wonder some of us get so "Americanized" in our talks, songs, lifestyles, and fashions. America is a successful, powerful and prosperous nation that attracts many people around the world, let alone our poor continent.

I mean we feel we must live like Americans: Eat like them, get jobs like them, earn a lot of dollars like them, be successful in our careers like them, attend nice schools, colleges and universities like them, make nice movies and music like them, become popular and famous like them, become smart and powerful like them. (Though we can't all prefer to raise our children like some of them.)

To paraphrase the above, I would like to say that we like a lot of Western stuff, but not all. This is obvious. Nobody likes everything in the other person from hair to toes. Just like you might have been fond of Michael Jackson but disliked his failure to appreciate who he was made to be. You might have been a great fanatic of Maradona but disliked his abuse of drugs. You might have appreciated Zinedine Zidane except for his vile reaction against Materazzi in the 2006 World Cup final. You may like the USA except for its interference in the private affairs of a sovereign state like Iraq. You might like Hitler's strategy for success but not his vision, or love your country but not its leadership. So, when given time, you may always point out something odd in the other person or the thing you're so fond of. Indeed we want Africa to get developed like the West, but not to become its copycat.

We're talking about a country that was once Malawi but wants to become Japan, a country that was DRC but must change into USA. Saying that is easy, but the doing is tough yet we can't do without. However, this is still my hope: Malawi can change into Japan, and DRC can become like the USA. I mean we can change, I see there's that potential and that's the feeling we all have. The question is: "Where do we go wrong, then? Is development really our dream?" If our answer to this question is "Yes," then a decade is more than enough for Africa to turn into a paradise. My own observation shows that we don't have even that desire at all. It's hard to explain why, but one can always find something substantial on which to base his argument.

Based on the management of our countries, one can easily conclude that many of our leaders don't have the desire to change our countries. It's such a big shame, but that's how the majority of them really manage our countries.

I'm a citizen of a nation that marked its independence in 1960 (several decades now since the so-called "oppressors" stepped out), but the country looks no different from hell. At least those we viewed as "oppressors" and constantly referred to as "imperialists" managed to leave some traces behind that help my country to score the "next to last" position on the continent's ranking, even today.

Since Caucasians stepped out of my country in 1960 there's nothing concrete happening. It has been moving backward at an amazing pace. I mean *nothing*—it's no exaggeration and I don't know any other English word that can properly describe it. Yet I don't have to use some euphemism in this matter. "Nothing" is the only word to describe what is happening in my country. That country is being managed like nobody's business. Things are progressing from bad to worse. So many people know what I'm talking about. In fact, it would be a sin to use any other word than "nothing" to describe the condition of DRC. What can you say of a country where you have no guarantee of electricity for domestic use in the presence of the great power supply of the Inga hydroelectric facility, which is being used effectively even by some other African countries? A country that has no traffic lights even in its overcrowded capital city—and the very cartoon-fashioned ones do not function because of excessive power cuts? A country where members of the defense force, police, teachers, and other public services do not know if they will be paid at month's end? A place where universities and so-called public schools do not have even facilities as basic as toilets? A naturally rich nation with not even a single airplane allowed to fly outside the continent? A nation where a computer in a public office is seen as an outstanding achievement in this twenty-first century? A country where the unique up-to-standard soccer stadium gets rehabilitated only after several warnings of a ban from FIFA? The worst for me is that no town in DRC is linked to another by an asphalt road.

I know when you meet an ignorant Congolese national and challenge him on such issues he would deny this truth and even label me a foreigner or something worse. The type of citizens who think that hiding or advocating for the evils of their leaders means being loyal citizens are only found in Africa, and a great number is in DRC. I look at those fellow compatriots with so much contempt because their denial of facts make our irresponsible leaders sink even more comfortably in their chairs. The truth is: Africans, especially my fellow Congolese, suffer from "identity syndrome." And so they have chosen to defend their identity with their expensive clothes, their famous music and fanciful talks, especially when they're in the presence of strangers.

It's irritating to see nothing progressing in a country as resource-rich as DRC. That's unbelievable. Congolese citizens respond to the poor service delivery by their government by deserting their country. Some of us started deserting our country even long before the most recent tragic war broke out. One of our attitudes that make me sick is the fact of denying that our country fails to offer even basic services to its population, especially in the presence of strangers. And we think that playing the devil's advocate to our leaders' wrongs and our countries' inability to make any progress means being loyal to one's country. Unfortunately, that's the opposite.

I believe we can easily get our message across when we start sharing our stories with our caring neighbors instead of keeping on boasting about our nice music, expensive clothes, and our innumerable resources that only end up in the pockets of very, very few people. That won't get us any further. And anyway why would one play the devil's advocate? Our freedom comes from exposing our leaders' evils and recognizing that we need whatever resources they have stolen from us to rebuild our beautiful continent.

As I said earlier, DRC is moving backward at an incredible pace. A Congolese must confess the state of his country wherever he goes. And any other fellow African should never be impressed by fancy talks, expensive clothes, nice rumba music or anything else Congolese boast for, he must seek to help that dying nation. Every Congolese, including myself, should be challenged to make an effort to rebuild their country.

I was describing my country because I can't talk much about other countries but all I know is that the situation is almost the same in Africa. Maybe other countries' condition is the right answer to the question, "How would you describe hell if you were asked to?" I'm sorry if that's what's going on in your country. I don't want to interfere. That's why I would like to analyze the general situation of the continent based on my own country.

I know at this stage I must have caused the formation of two camps, but I must also try hard to get my way between the two, at least a moment sooner, before I get disturbed. Some critics in the opposite camp might say, "We doubt this guy is on this planet, especially on this continent. What does he expect our leaders to do after all these negative influences from outside? How does he expect us to get 'There' while we're being cunningly prevented (by Westerners, to be specific) from getting where we want to be? We're trying our best to make our first step, but always wars, exploitation of all kinds, apartheid, racism, and tribalism are pushed in to make everything crumble. Westerners would never let sleeping dogs alone. They're experts, so to speak, in interfering with other people's businesses and cleverly discouraging every good plan." I can identify with that, I used to utter such words. I unlearned it when I refused to accept it at face value. When I honestly decided to delve into these things, they proved to be wrong to me.

Yet, that is one possible criticism. I like criticism because it teaches you to keep cool under fire and it forms one's character in a great deal. That is yet another lesson our leaders fail to learn; they can't take criticism. They feel it "offends" their "right" to be "untouchable." What a tragedy! Let's hope this is just one of the diseases of infancy that is likely to disappear when we become adults. I believe when we become adults in the next century we won't get mad at somebody who gently reproaches us for having used money for a wrong shopping list when we purchased our items than it is to be advised not to use a red pen in correspondence.

But if one takes the trouble to analyze the above criticism, the whole bundle of sentences would be summarized into something like: "As long as there's a Western world on the other side, Africa will never develop. *Never*, full stop." This implies that Africa must stop budgeting for development and put that word off their mind. It has no chance to get any further, it must just forget about development or any of its implications. Unfortunately, that's exactly the opposite of what I have in my mind. I meant it when I said, "Malawi can become like Japan and DRC can look like USA." That criticism may be based on fear or lack of confidence, perhaps an inferiority complex or low self-esteem.

Should we believe that the biggest hindrance to our development is the presence of Western countries forcing us to take up weapons and start up wars to destroy all we have? Should we believe they are the sowers of this hatred going on among the members of our different ethnic groups? They're forcing us to set up mining companies to get them diamonds? Should this be taken to mean that in order for Africa to appear on the world map

Europe and America should disappear (or vice versa)? Or rather Africa cannot be clearly seen on the same map where Europe and America appear? None of that is really convincing. We must learn to stop blaming others for our own mess. We must avoid shifting responsibilities; that's a sign of immaturity. When one becomes a good actor he learns how to carefully play well the unique role he has in the scene. He knows that, no matter how short or insignificant might his role seem, it has a big impact on the entire scene and affects the whole play. And so, in every role we play in the scene of life, we must be careful how we handle it. That's wisdom. If the West is behind every war in Africa, rousing every hatred among our tribes, backing every mismanagement of our resources, racism, and all other vices, then I should admit they're the most difficult people to live with on this planet. But I personally avoid shifting responsibilities or imputing everyone else in my own mess. Even though I'm aware of some of their quasi-intolerable wrongs, I don't think they deserve such blame for our own evils. And, after all, it's now almost fifty years since some of our countries achieved independence, and the reason for our underdevelopment should still be colonization? What about Malaysia? What of Israel, after surviving years of holocaust and anti-Semitism? What about other nations in Asia and South America that were also colonized and marked their independence almost at the same time with our countries? We are not on the same pace of development with these nations at all. How so? After half a century of independence we have nothing to show off other than what Europeans left; and the irony is that we are not even able to maintain what they left. What an irresponsible race we are!

It's hard for some of us to endorse what I'm about to say, but it needs a lot of introspection: I'm inclined to think that even if nothing like colonization (what we view as interference) had happened, some of the most awful crimes we commit everyday in Johannesburg, atrocities we perpetrate in Darfur, genocide we authored in Rwanda, and cannibalism practices recorded in DRC for self-enrichment and the search for power, would have occurred anyway. And if Westerners are behind some of these things then they must be taking advantage of our corrupt character: our greed, our "inborn" hatred, our selfish ambitions and our domineering attitude. I'm not sure whether Westerners make us greedy and selfish or they find us so. If they turn us into such devil-like people (I mean if they smartly turn us greedy and selfish and fill our minds with domineering attitudes), then we know, at least now, that we should use our brains smartly. We have to dare to be ourselves, and that would help us quench their schemes.

But if they find us already corrupt to the core, then the task we have is that of rebuilding our society—and this time the structure must go deep, really. C. S. Lewis remarked, when you wear blue spectacles everything else you look at will turn blue. The task is ours to take off or change the spectacles. By so doing we'd be able to prevent any outsider from manipulating us in future.

If Westerners are so crooked that they can easily bait even those of us who are not interested in becoming presidents or prime ministers, or in getting rich at the expense of others, then we must consider the following. Suppose you're the head of a family. What would you do if someone handed you weapons and ordered you to kill your kids (those little ones you love so dearly), to slay your partner (the one you'd rather not live without), to hand over your wealth (that you acquired from your hard work or inherited), to hate and sacrifice your relatives and friends (those you believe are giving any meaning to your life at all). If you find the answer, go and apply it.

But if even the needle of our free will watch can still be easily influenced to point west, then our hope is only in the coming centuries. And I doubt if we will fare well even in the next centuries because the brainy mind today is likely to be brainier tomorrow and the brainiest forever—but also the most deceitful, fraudulent and cunning if it chooses to. If the war we're in is that of minds, then we have to work very hard to sharpen our minds because the sharper they are, the more we stand the chance to reverse the situation. Fortunately—and I believe this beyond any doubt—the war we have to wage has got less to do with minds. This is what we have to dodge to concentrate on our strengths and do what we can without bothering much about our neighbors' minds.

We must always remember that "the man who hands out the gun and the one who pulls the trigger to shoot are equally perpetrators." Both should be apprehended whenever something bad happens, and they're both to be called in if people want to find a durable solution to the problem. This is simply to mean that the West that we think is behind most of the evils happening on our continent today and those of us who execute their plans on the continent are equally wrong. All of them should be apprehended if we need to get a durable solution to the problem.

# Chapter Two

# What Lies Behind Civil Wars

Well, at issue here is "unwillingness." Some African leaders are not ready to do what is expected of them or do what they've promised. The driving force behind all this is "lack of love." I believe the second breeds the first. Lack of love causes unwillingness: It's quite impossible to do something for the people you don't love, unless you want to offer a fake service. Lack of love is the root of so many evils on our continent. Interesting enough, Africa is the only continent where solidarity is intensely observed and chatted about, this should be just another way of manifesting and promoting hypocrisy in an uncovered manner. But I don't think we really need to encourage hypocrisy in any way.

And apart from what we call solidarity, I can hardly think of anything else that could evidently demonstrate active love in Africa. So if solidarity fails to prove active love, then I reckon it wouldn't sound strange if someone said there's no active mutual love in Africa. I think we still need more sermons on love. It's a nice topic, anyway. It's not only nice but the foundation of every human relationship if one really means to keep them firm.

Let's quickly recap what we said in the first chapter: The West is bringing weapons to initiate war in Liberia, or is it simply our desire to get rich through diamond that turns us into devils? Should we blame the West for our fellow brothers who were tortured and mutilated in Sierra Leone or it's simply our greed for natural resources and hunger for worthless power?

Who caused genocide in Rwanda if not the two tribes (Hutu and Tutsi) consumed with either achieving or preserving power? Who is causing millions of innocents to lose their lives in DRC if not its neighbors driven by the desire to get Congolese natural resources to become wealthy or perhaps powerful? Should we blame Westerners for all this? No way. This is our own fault.

Perhaps I'm trying to overlook some facts that have been acknowledged by many. But my point remains that the world superpowers might offer weapons and other required technologies to incite us to wage wars against each other so they can get our resources, but who implement their plans? They play with our perception of power and wealth. They know very well that for most of our leaders a strong army is the one that attacks its neighboring countries. They know that African heads of state think that being powerful means conquering other people's lands. Our leaders like it when they pile up countless money in Swiss or Luxembourg banks (or any other banks in Western countries), though it gets frozen after they step down or when they die. Westerners know that's what our leaders like the most, and that's the climax of our thinking.

Certainly, for such a spoiled race weapons would be supplied in exchange with mines, oil, money or anything else that is at stake. Of course, that should be the simplest formula. When Westerners need these commodities (and we know how badly they seek after them) they wouldn't care much whether other people die in the process or not. They wouldn't care whether these resources are taken illegally, looted, or stolen from other countries. But they don't put any of our villages ablaze, they don't mutilate our children, they don't rape our women and girls, they don't force our ten-year-old boys to join the army, and they don't pull the trigger of any machine gun to shoot our old schoolmates or our childhood friends. They do nothing inhumane. Perhaps they know at this time of the world's history one should strive to respect someone else's rights; but yet they know some crazy neighbors whose conscience never know how to distinguish good from bad whenever power or wealth is offered. I'm told that some people or some ethnic groups amongst us are very smart, but I've never seen any such sign. Those of us who are admired for their intelligence are the great violators of human rights and the worst perpetrators of many atrocities on the continent. That questions their intelligence. If being clever means the ability to attack other countries to achieve wealth or organize mass killing, especially of your own race in order to achieve power, then I'm left with no definition of what being clever means.

There's no need to blame anybody else for what happens in Africa. We are the authors of all that which staggers every inhabitant of this planet. We're at the center of every war being waged on our own continent. As President Obama said, for too many Africans conflict is part of life as constant as the sun. And this has made Africa the crude caricature of a continent at perpetual war.

I can only accept that Westerners are at the center of the black man's misery in Africa if I see people of white skin in uniform from somewhere in the West standing in the front lines issuing orders on the battlefields. But, unfortunately, all I've seen involved in such bloody games are those bloodthirsty fellows of my own skin color (from my continent or even hired from other continents) so caught up in radical selfish ambitions and so consumed with hatred.

I had received some criticism on this point sometimes back. The critic said that everything we see happening is played behind the scene. What we see or those we see aren't the ones really involved in the game. But this criticism always gave me some break and hope that we're not far from stopping wars. My confidence is based on my experience as a trained actor.

When I was acting at university, my lecturer and my directors used to encourage us to improvise on stage. If Westerners play it behind the scenes and we're the ones on the field or going up on stage, so to speak, then we have all the time in our hands to change their plans. To improvise. But to such corrupt people like us, improvisation is the last thought on our minds. Therefore, whatever happens on the field happens because we allow it, so to speak. And if some crazy things happen on the field, that would be our own fault; we shouldn't blame anybody else for that. We must choose to do what is favorable to our continent. We must choose to improvise for our own welfare. We must choose to deliberately ignore any other deceitful advice from behind the scene—we have that power to change everything when we're left alone on the field.

So, the lecturer was seemingly saying, "I've taught you the skills, but I'm not with you on stage. You're on your own." Yet, she was the one behind the scene. That urge would mean freedom to actors. And we always put that advice into practice. We would deliberately change the text and use our own words, and sometimes change the props as we found fit. There was nothing wrong with that. Yet the truth is this, even if she wouldn't have said anything, she knew as we also did, that since we're alone on stage (on the field) we would not stick to *all* her instructions. Even in soccer, especially during penalty shootouts, many coaches tell players, "Now you're alone. Use your skills."

One thing I like about somebody playing behind the scene is that he seems to be clearly telling the person on the field: "You must use your mind properly. I know you're able to handle this situation correctly. I don't want to manipulate or dictate you, and I can't even if I choose to. Be alone!" And if we're being influenced from behind the scene to kill each other then our brains are the object of utter mockery.

Even though winning is what a team is in for, the player or actor can sometimes choose to make everything fall apart. He can choose to lose or make the whole play unsuccessful, depending on his personal reasons. A player or an actor can choose to sabotage his coach or his director or whoever is behind the scene for reasons that are known to him alone. And he can only succeed to play such a tricky game because he's alone on the field. The fact of being alone on the scene allows this gaffe or sabotage to happen because on the ground, the coach can't interfere anymore and all his orders behind the scene are of no use if the player refuses to consider them. And in our own case, we must choose to ignore anyone behind the scene (if there's any at all), to secure our continent. We have to make up our minds now and stop rehearsing and performing exactly the same text or using the same props when we get on stage because there (on stage) we're left on our own to decide what to do. If we fail to do that, then we're the authors of our own suffering. And in reality, that's who we are. No one else, in fact, should be expected to defend our case, not even the international community. And we shouldn't blame anyone for our present condition.

I would like to prevent some of my readers from asking one question. From the previous chapter I have a feeling that some of you are being tempted to ask: Why are we made of such rotten stuff that we can't even stand on our own and resist outside influences? That's what we shouldn't ask because, as was remarked by C.S. Lewis, "The better stuff a creature is made of—the cleverer and stronger and freer it is—then the better it will be if it goes right but also the worse it will be if it goes wrong." So, to have a better mind does not guarantee that things will work perfectly well.

Now some of us can see why I kept on saying we must stop blaming or imputing others in our own mistakes. We have a role to play in everything that happen to us and so it's up to us rather to play it in a clever way. The ball is in our camp when we're alone on the scene, so to speak, and the task is ours to play it right.

Yet I must suggest some practical way of dealing with this scenario, and it's what I can contribute if I'm asked to stop atrocities in Africa. It may sound very simplistic to some but I have to say it anyway: "I'll refuse any weapons handed to me." At this point I'm aware that I'd be told "It's easy to say it, but putting it into practice when it becomes a reality is not as easy as you think." This offer, we're told, is always accompanied with money and other advantages. I also must admit this is the toughest brainteaser one could ever face. But, should one accept weapons to start war, killing his fellow countrymen in order to get money and power in return? Should I sacrifice millions of my compatriots' lives to achieve power and wealth? Should I start up a war so I can be appointed or appoint myself in one of the highest positions in my state or become wealthy?

Quite bluntly (and this really would make sense to many) only a fool can do that. Only some people of rotten stuff can accept such a filthy offer. It's only cranks who can accept to play such a bloody game. This act easily reveals what substance one's mind is made of. Four strong and clear proofs of "selfish ambitions" can be drawn out of it: killing your fellow countrymen for "dead ends;" failure to willingly lay down your *life* to spare your fellows' *lives*; greed for material prosperity and self-enrichment; and domineering spirit: hunger for power.

In any life we live and in any society we're part of, we ought to be unselfish for many good reasons. I've got no time to go through all of them, but you'd agree with me that one of the characters—in your neighbor or perhaps your friend—that makes you sick is selfishness. You can't wait for seconds to see them going on selfish before you exclaim, "It's not fair."

So, I get the offer, I refuse and resist it. And immediately when we're informed that such an offer is around, we must appoint a secret agency to initiate propaganda for sabotage. The information must flow as fast as a bullet, and it must reach everyone within few hours like oil upon the waters. This could prepare every one of us who is approached for the same offer to stand his ground. And so on. It's even when true solidarity is needed. I believe unity is only strength when people can see, perceive, and act the same way.

There's an old fable of two buffalos that remained indomitable because they ate, walked, lived, talked, suggested, handled issues, defended, stood, made decisions and saw their interests together. That's the right illustration for unity and solidarity. That's truly walking hand in hand as humans without necessarily seeing eye to eye.

I wonder why we should talk about African solidarity and unity only when it comes to sharing food, and attending funerals in big numbers while we can easily kill or contribute to the destruction of one another whenever given the offer of power, bank notes and pieces of diamonds. To me, and I believe to so many other people here in Africa, this doesn't make any sense at all, especially in this century. I can hardly think of any normal person who kills his parents, relatives and friends just for money and some other funny promises from his neighbors. We should think win-win because the world has enough for everyone to shine. Yet Africans have always been great subscribers to win-lose. They do not hesitate to kill millions to get one man rich. Now I know that by the time we get twenty millionaires we shall be left only with heaps of burned rubbles around the continent. Shame on us!

That's how heartless we are. Where is our love? Where's our solidarity? Sadly, some of those who sign such contracts sometimes die in the process of trying to cash their checks or getting their diamonds to the right markets. Often some tricky games are played in this business and double-crossing is the most frequent one. So many African leaders who stored up their wealth in Western countries found their money frozen in those banks after stepping down or when they died. Others have never had any access to that money at all. And, ironically, those who are thought to be supporting such atrocities at first are the ones who accuse them of such carnage and order their money to be frozen. And in the end all the money is lost, nothing is gained. Unfortunately, none of our leaders has drawn any lesson from that sad experience so far. What a tragedy! I wonder from which world all those hard-headed African fellows come.

My fellow Africans disappoint me to the point of making me believe that all the people I see dying in Hollywood and Bollywood action movies are real people, dying literally. Anyway, I've never been in Hollywood or

Bollywood to doubt about people dying in their movies. The reality of war in Africa would make someone believe everything portrayed in those action movies. Just as an actor of Hollywood toys around with people's lives, it's what we're witnessing in Africa every day. We've all become movie stars. Sometimes, it seems that the number of actors and victims we see in all action movies is exactly the same we see in reality every day in Africa. I have no doubt some of us have been taking up the proper names of Hollywood and Bollywood stars so to enjoy the scenes they're playing in Liberia, Sierra Leone, Congo Brazzaville, DRC, Burundi, Rwanda, Cote D'Ivoire and Uganda's Hollywoods. That's more than savagery. That's showing how primitive we are, even in such an advanced world like ours. Does all this really happen in the name of change or liberation as often claimed? Or it's simply dollar and power mania? We've turned Africa into hell—a world where people's lives are getting cheaper than bank notes and power. How could we, even in this twenty-first century, still be consumed with such petty things?

Suppose someone supports what I suggested earlier: "They offer you weapons, and you refuse them"—I guess the possible retort would be: What if somebody else accepts them? This is a true expression of doubt and concern over one's life. Some would quickly anticipate a conclusion: "I won't be spared," or "I'll certainly get shot." At this level one may think of another possible reason for accepting the offer, I mean the offer for weapons for mass destruction—and not any other mass but his fellow countrymen: safety. And this could be a mistake, because weapons in anyone's hands can either be protective or self-destructive.

Those taking up weapons for protection often think: "If I don't accept them—or, perhaps, if I don't set myself in a good position to execute others first—someone else may accept them and shoot me first. To safeguard my life or to avoid any kind of oppression, I must accept the offer." Such decision may be based on this line of reasoning: "I should control them. I should dominate them, not vice versa." A domineering attitude is back again.

Insecure? Want to save your life? Unfortunately, sometimes in the violent attempt to save his life with weapons, one may tragically lose it; conversely, in the endeavour to willingly sacrifice it, one may amazingly save it. Life is full of surprises. Often it works exactly the opposite way. That experience taught me not to waste much time thinking how to save or secure my life because it's seemingly being taken care of on a much higher level. But I know it would be strange if I expected everyone else to share the same belief with me. That's being an elitist; I don't want to be one.

Most frequently, we try to save our lives with our own weapons (swords, guns, missiles, and all); this often proves to be a failure. I know some mighty nations that were destroyed despite all their sophisticated weapons. I remember some powerful countries that failed to neutralize their enemies' network despite their mighty intelligence and advanced technology. Others were easily fragmented into smaller pieces despite their powerful intelligence and weaponry. Some of you may agree with me that life is not easy to protect with one's weapon; it may look easy, but it's hard. Success in such an attempt is not guaranteed despite all the weapons one may employ. Trying to save one's life is similar to appointing other people to guard you. The irony in it is that they can't even successfully protect their own lives; how much can they be trusted to protect another person's life? What I'm trying to say is that none of us can manage to save or secure his life in the true sense of the word. I'm not talking about self-help or self-defense. That's another story. I also wish all of us would learn some martial arts for self-defence; but protecting one's life in the true sense transcends our ability.

But we must know our true enemy. When you know your enemy, you're likely to understand his mind, how he works over his plans, and what his strategy would be. Our enemies are those who offer us weapons and incite us behind the scenes to start wars. Now our task is to try to scrupulously study them in order to know their strategy. We're probably going to win in the next encounter because then we shall be able to quench their schemes after discovering their strategy.

When one kills his fellow countrymen and even family members, he's immediately creating an atmosphere of insecurity around himself—even with those who trusted him the most. Everybody else would soon be thinking: "Now that he's in control of military hardware and doesn't hesitate to silence even his own relatives, he can possibly fire anyone else who gets on his way." And that's the case with some African tyrants like Mobutu, Idi Amin, El Bashir, and others. What is left here is far from what might be called leadership.

So, the more cruel one becomes, the more people get scared of him—even his closest friends and relatives would keep a distance. No one would trust him, not even his own children. I would rather challenge us to think in terms of "our welfare" in order to save "our lives." When you succeed in securing other people's lives, you're likely to be secured among them. One's safety is best guaranteed in a group rather than in singleness.

Unfortunately, the majority of us still need a strong remedy to neutralize the "individualism syndrome" in them. "Me" in Africa tends to become more important than "Him." It even extends beyond "Them.". So "'I' alone matter, they can all disappear." This has become a contagious and deadly disease killing millions of innocents on this continent. It killed thousands in Liberia, Uganda, Burundi, Cote D'Ivoire, Sierra Leone, and Congo Brazzaville. It killed millions in Rwanda, DRC, and Angola in pursuit of money and power. What a pity! Money and power are the driving force behind "I," instigating him to open fire to his fellow brothers, sisters, and even parents. "I" simply opens fire, not caring who takes the bullet, as long as money or power is achieved. That's how confused we have become on this continent.

In conclusion, we must be careful to make any mistake here. If someone thinks that stopping enticing "Mr. I" with power and money would be the right strategy to end war, he may be right but he could be missing another important point. If there's anyone who thinks we must stop foreign countries from exporting their weapons to Africa and that would be the end of wars on the continent, I will tell him what it is like: It's like trying to stop your friends from picking up whores from streets. It's more like a shop trying to warn its customers not to buy its expired products while all its gates are still open. Or, like a mother who earnestly attempts to get toast off her kitchen while she carries on buying breads. I mean none of this is to be done before the other. It's like the law of offer and demand. The demand is present that's why there's an offer, likewise the offer is made because of demand.

This is to say that if anyone wants to stop his friends from getting prostitutes from streets, he should—in the meantime—attempt to stop prostitutes from standing by streets. He should target the two groups at once. Any supermarket manager desiring to prevent his customers from buying expired products from his shop needs to close all the gates of his shop or take off all the expired items as soon as the advertisement goes to advertising companies. And a mother who would like to get toast off her kitchen should stop buying breads altogether.

Therefore, any peace activist willing to stop other countries from "illegally" exporting weapons to Africa must make sure he stops all the buyers (in this case, both power-hungry folks and rebels) of his country from seeking them. These two processes should go together. I would rather say, stopping "Mr. I" from *focusing* too much on money and power would be another way of waving goodbye to this ugly short word—war.

Consequently, "Mr. I" must be taught not to be so anxious about *his* welfare, because *our* welfare is more meaningful. Now, I guess we're getting what I've been trying to point out in this chapter. Instead of wasting time thinking that his safety is at risk if he refuses weapons, it's better to think, "I, one individual, would rather die instead of millions of my fellow compatriots." This is sacrifice for Africa's sake. I mean, instead of thinking, "What if another person accepts those weapons?" you should plead to your God (if you believe in one at all) that he shouldn't accept them too, for his country's sake. And whenever the next person is approached and given the offer, he must respond the same: "I refuse them for my country's sake." Guess the result if everyone goes on answering like that to the very last. We'd quickly change the AU anthem to joyfully and proudly sing a new one: "Africa will be number one on the finish line to getting paradise."

# Chapter Three

# Should It Be Leading Or Dealing?

In so many African countries, age is still a problem in politics. I know a country where the president was not easily accepted by the political veterans of his country simply because he was still young (in his early thirties). His age was a big problem to them. But when I learned about the age at which those veterans got involved into politics, I found out that many of them were still very young as well. The president was referred to as a teenager without any convincing reasons.

My question still is, if that young man was seen to be too young to rule the country, with whom, then, were they comparing him? I would accept that he was young if they compared him with their sons and daughters, for example, but compared to other former leaders who once occupied some senior government positions in that country or other countries in Africa, the young man was mature enough to rule—just as they saw themselves mature and capable enough when they joined politics.

My appeal to fellow Africans is that, wherever we are, we should stop stagnating on such nonsense. They're delaying our progress. Anybody holding onto that assumes to be mature, experienced and wiser than the younger—like a father, for instance. And the first responsibility of a father is to help his child become mature and develop the sense of responsibility that he needs to manage any leadership position later. A father must make sure that his son learns to do the right things so he reflects him. When the father starts doubting his son—complaining that he can't make it—he's immediately revealing the level of his own irresponsibility because he's merely saying, "I've failed to bring the best out of my son." In other words, he's afraid that his son might only bring shame on his family's name. In order to cover that shame and failure (I think it's a failure to educate), he thinks it's better to stop him from assuming any important position before he's known to be part of his family. Anyone who tells me that his full-grown son can't make it is probably telling me to stop trusting him as well.

(Any angel's child is an angel and any demon's child is a demon. Any angel's child would be expected to be angelic, just like any demon's child would be expected to be demonic. An angel can't bear a demon, and likewise a demon can't bear an angel. As the saying goes: Like father like son.)

Stop doubting your child if you really know who you are and what you can do. Trust him. Wish him all the best. Give him all the support he needs to become what he should be: a responsible and capable man, a successful leader.

To paraphrase the above, I would like to say the following: Age is not a problem. I believe in this case one's attitude could be a big problem. If one knows how much he invested in his child he'd never doubt or undermine him. He'd rather be proud of him, especially when he assumes some higher position in the government, and he should be ready and willing to support him at any cost so he doesn't bring him any shame. If you think you're old and wise enough, and you really trust your own wisdom, your experience and expertise then offer to be your leader's personal advisor. Give what you believe is worth. Help him work as you would—for your own benefit, or corporate benefit at least.

So the first time one learns that his leader is a teenager and he doubts his leadership skills, then the next and perhaps the wisest step he can ever make could be to help and support him—not to seek how he would brutally substitute him. After all, I personally don't think there would be any problem if the matter were to rule or lead only. But if the matter becomes: "This young man is going to get rich now that he assumes that position," then there would be a big problem that may easily result in an armed conflict. And, in so many instances, that's the case in Africa.

Yet another problem we're facing today is of leaders refusing to step down once they get into those offices. Once a leader gets elected or appoints himself through violence, he becomes so consumed with preserving the power and even starts manipulating the people who helped him climb the ladder. He starts by changing the entire structure of the country through amendments. He tries to adjust the law to work in his favour, and then he turns the country into a kingdom (in his mind, and on his hidden draft first) even though it may still be a republic or a sovereign state on the original documents. Yet, to quote president Obama, history is not on the side of those who use coups to achieve power or change constitutions to maintain it.

There's a Swahili proverb that says: "You can see clearly during the day while the sun is still shining. In the darkness of night you can barely see anything." This proverb, when used in politics, could mean: "It's not easy to do something now that you didn't accomplish in other terms—no matter how long you try to prolong your terms. They probably won't help you. It's your night already. So, give chance to someone else whose sight is not yet affected by darkness. He stands the chance to succeed because he still has a 'sharp vision'." But he must also be tired of seeing his country or continent in the last row on the development line.

I mean whoever comes to power foolishly thinks he's a successor of such and such a fictitious king from such and such a fictitious kingdom. He views the state house as a private domain where nobody else can ever get. He gets so much in love with the state house that he can't leave it for someone else. He wants the rulings and decisions to be his alone as long as he lives. He's after power but, more than anything else, he wants to control. What self-absorption!

In 2007, President Paul Biya of Cameroon imposed a law that allows the head of state to contend as many times as he wishes. Lives were lost in the process of silencing those who oppose the idea. Though already one of the long-serving heads of state in Africa, President Biya endlessly sought to convince parliamentarians to pass the bill that would give him more years in the office. And he seemed unmindful of the implications this could have on his country.

And, as was once observed by a Namibian political analyst, Dr. Joseph Diescho, "Africa has borne and continues to bear a heavy burden because of this short-sightedness and small mindedness of political elites who command that, because they're in power at a particular time—as Chinua Achebe would put it—all disagreement should cease and the whole people must speak with a single voice."

He starts considering everybody else as mere employees at his service. In some African governments, some people are viewed like robot machines: They're not even supposed to talk.

In the management of state affairs, there seems to be a line drawn somewhere that only the leader himself knows where it starts and where it ends; anyone else trying to go or do beyond that line is punished severely or dismissed from the system immediately. We're playing the politics of "hidden policies" in Africa. And the bad side of such policies is that you wouldn't know what they imply and so you would easily fall into the trap. As a result, anyone trying to go or do beyond his assigned tasks is sent off immediately. There, tribalism comes in. The whole tendency is to turn everything into a dynasty. The leader starts feeling that the state should have been a kingdom and the state house a palace, a place where his children, concubines, and relatives would never depart from. He feels he must protect, preserve and reinforce "their family supremacy" before he dies. He finally turns it into a kingdom-like at last.

Unfortunately, as observed by Diescho, the political analyst I quoted earlier, "The uninformed notion of one nation, one leader, one thought is perilous. We should always remember that diversity of views nourishes a sustainable democratic and even economic system. Some political regimes have imposed one thought upon the people and stifled individual voices and that have led to the imminent collapse of the same systems. So it is a waste of time trying to feed up those systems."

It becomes compulsory to concur with any leader's decisions no matter how silly they may be. No criticism. But if one can accept a compliment, why shouldn't he take a criticism, too? No more work follow-ups in the leader's office. A few days before his death, President Omar Bongo of Gabon ordered the detention of five anti-corruption campaigners for having disclosed that he buys French properties with the proceeds of corruption. That's the leadership syndrome in Africa. Anything the leader does, thinks, or says should automatically become perfect and deserve the strongest and longest applause. All other people are rendered to the status of children. What a leadership misconception!

If his tribe was small, he would encourage them to deliberately ignore family planning chats. If they were not in the army, they'd be forced to join. If they were not well educated or sometimes not even interested in formal education at all, they'd be forced to enroll in all learning institutions, even with fake or unsatisfactory qualifications. Even if they were not willing to work, they'd be forced to. And all these are simply "maintain the power" strategies. Well, these encouragements and exhortations are favourable for any development, but they may only be useful if they're all aimed at promoting every other citizen in the country instead of a specific tribe or clan. That would be the best and most successful propaganda for development. As was remarked by President Obama, in this twenty-first century only capable, reliable, and transparent institutions are the key to success. And so long as we're unable to forge such institutions, we cannot talk of development.

Unfortunately, in the regimes we have been describing, other tribes are considered like intruders, and only those who befriend or totally submit stand the chance to be accommodated. The rest suffer terribly. Funny enough, they're also patiently waiting for their turn to retaliate and do even worse. Every other tribe that gets the power later targets the "big fish for their baskets" and works with: "you must also feel the heat" attitude—that of resentment. And usually they grab that power between "the lion's teeth." And so it becomes an unending vicious circle.

Ironically, they spend all their time and money inventing some formulas to achieve power. They use every means possible to achieve it: rebellion, opposition or even coups. Frankly, what we feel when we crave for power is not supposed to be called hunger at all, it's more than hunger. Sometimes one can bear hunger even if it is driving him crazy or robbing him of all strength but it's not so with power. What you can't bear is to see the other person seated on the throne. That's the exact picture of Africa. Even while I'm typing this sentence, some of us are conspiring to throw others out, not necessarily because they've identified some holes in their philosophies, but simply because they want to be seen on the thrones, too. They may not literally take up guns to fight but there's more than gun-shooting going on every day in our countries. I wouldn't be surprised to hear that some crazy things happened somewhere else on the continent even a few minutes before this book is submitted for printing. This is predictable on the continent. What an unfortunate position we are in! I don't think I would favor politics if its prime focus were to search for thrones as it is in Africa.

I believe tribalism is the source of most of these problems. And it comes in as result of pride (some tribes viewing themselves as being special or superior than others), selfishness (some tribes viewing themselves as the only rightful owners of the country's wealth), revenge (some tribes feeling like they're excluded from the system), inferiority or superiority complex (some tribes viewing themselves as smaller or inferior, while others considering themselves to be bigger and superior). If we are wise, we should seek to nurture diversity. It must be the source of our strength, not the cause of our division.

Remember, none of us is a peak at all. I mean none of us, including those seated on the throne today, is the embodiment of wisdom. When one sees millions of fellow citizens around, he should view them as potential leaders. We're surrounded by people who can do greater than we hardly think of them. Yet that is what we either willingly or unwillingly refuse to acknowledge in Africa.

If you're a leader today, don't ever be afraid of those around you. Their success shouldn't be a scarecrow to you; it should rather be the object of your delight. Entrust them with as many responsibilities as possible. Draw them closer. Help them develop the feeling of belonging—to their country, not to your kingdom—it could stop them from mismanaging the public treasure. The moment you stop trusting them, they will start feeling insecure and fearing they might be dismissed at any time. And this is when they get their wake-up calls, so to speak, and as a result theft, corruption, and mismanagement follow. Indeed, they'd steal as much as they can before they are dismissed. Consequently, poor, innocent, ordinary men fall victims.

We need to develop another leadership style giving everybody a better chance to benefit and contribute to his country with all his ability. Everyone is a citizen and must be treated equally. Amazingly enough, that's found in all our constitutions: "All people are equal before the law." Now, unless we're cheating on each other, every single article in our constitutions must be obeyed. That's why we make them, after all.

"Putting the right people in the right positions" is yet another important formula that could help us eliminate all the differences between our tribes. It won't be long before we realize that it's not only people from one tribe who are the right people for all the key positions we have in the country. Those who could practice putting the right people in the right positions would quickly notice how it tremendously breaks all those tribal differences in all the strata of the community. We must always bear to heart that we wouldn't be marketing our continent at all if all we do is to reward those who don't possess the ability to sell the continent and push aside those who can. By putting the right people in the right positions, we're likely to get everyone involved into the system. The more we practice it, the more our countries are likely to advance. And beyond all else, we must always remember that we're not dealing, we're leading. So, let's get up there and lead!

# Chapter Four

# 80/20 Percent Business

This was the most challenging chapter for me. I had to think twice before I could include it among the chapters of this book. The difficult part of it wasn't because I had run out of ideas, but because I always avoid to present something that would appear to be an *a priori* conclusion or something that would sound like a fact yet simple rumours. In fact, one of my favorite sayings is, "I hate nobody—but anybody whose speeches, statements and beliefs are based on assumptions and prejudices annoys me the most." And so I felt I would end up in the trap I've been avoiding in my whole life, and which I would never like to even find myself in. I found myself squeezed. But, specifically for this one, I also thought that rumors can sometimes be interesting to some, and for such people it would be unfair to leave this out simply because it sounded untrue to me. I finally decided to reproduce the whole story as it was presented to me. Whether you'll take it as a rumor still or as a fact, it's none of my concern. Nevertheless, I still hold that some rumors have some truth in them or are closer to the truth or based on the truth. Just like the old adage goes, "There's no smoke without fire."

Now these rumors are hitting the streets of Africa every day. But I wouldn't be surprised if some of us haven't heard anything about them. It's only the law of human nature (knowing right and wrong) that you'd expect everybody else to be aware of because that is built inside every one of us. But any other information that comes from outside requires someone's chance, so to speak, to come across it. I should admit that it bugged me so much that I decided to open my ears lest it make me sick. Can't wait to know what 80/20 percent business is all about, right? Just like myself.

It was summarized to me in the following words: "In order to maintain their power, some African leaders are forced to sacrifice eighty percent of their resources (especially mines and oil) to other countries and remain with twenty percent only." What a blatant loss! I exclaimed. To run a business that maximizes one hundred percent of profit, and then share that profit in two unequal parts: the producer (business owner) gets twenty percent and the associate (business partner) gets eighty percent.

Not even a Good Samaritan can accept such a loss. If that's true, I suppose you'd also like to know from which planet are those countries just as I did. You can't easily accept that to have been happening on our planet, let alone our poor continent, could you?

For the first time, I just didn't agree and exclaimed in shock, "What on earth is that business here for?" I objected that it can't happen on earth just as you're also feeling right now, I guess. Of course, it's totally hard to allow that to enter your mind. And you can notice how it's difficult even for me to get the right words to explain it. It's really an awful scenario, if it exists.

On the other hand, after this was frequently chatted about among my fellow countrymen (I came across all this after the second war broke out in my country in 1998), I came to give it a nod, and of course, looked at it with a different eye. But I never stopped wondering what that loss could be if such business was being run somewhere in Africa. I never stopped asking myself why countries in such an indescribable state of poverty like ours should get involved in such business. However, I thought to myself, if that business really exists, I would encourage the "associate" business partner to carry on doing it because if there should be any business to run at all, that's the right kind of it. Business means profit, anyway. These people should be the top and most successful businessmen we have in our world.

But, how many shares do they buy to get such a great deal of profit? The answer to that question seems to be blowing in the wind for the moment, perhaps we shall know it some times before it's too late for us. If this associate partner doesn't even labor for the business in question, then I have no qualm to confirm that he's beyond our material world. He must be from outside our material world, the rightful owner of everything around, up and underneath. So he takes eighty percent or he grabs nearly everything because it's his own property, so to speak.

There may be some objection at this level again. The possible objection to the above is that this businessman seems to be even more than anybody we can think of. Those of us who believe in the Bible know that the God of the Bible (though being the owner of everything as the Bible claims) doesn't seem to be so hard on the human race. He doesn't seem to be consumed with riches that way. He requests for ten percent only out of one hundred and doesn't take it anywhere out of anyone's reach. It's for the contributors' welfare. And he insists that it should be given willingly and cheerfully, not forcefully—meaning one has to give not under any pressure or oppression.

Amazingly enough, in some other religions' books, their gods don't even make any request on the followers' revenues. Yet they constantly show their generosity to their followers. If God is so tolerant of you and me in terms of giving (because he sees our state is so hopeless that we can't be charged that much), asking us to give only ten percent—and, for some of us, nothing—that we should give willingly not forcefully; who is this man getting at us mercilessly by using the opposite of God's practice? (It's clear that the supernatural is completely out of this business.) I think here we're dealing with some "Extrasupernatural man." And you and I can hardly think such a being exists.

Let's come back to the God of the Bible once more. (I don't want to preach, heaven knows.) He explains clearly why he takes the ten percent from our revenues. He demands it in order to recompense those who labour for him and also for charity purposes. But, honestly speaking, I think for God this wouldn't be the only reason behind his urge to give. I think the essence for his request would be to test and teach his people about generosity, which is one of the greatest values of humanity and key to abundance.

Why should this stranger take all that big amount of stuff? No answer can ever be given to that question with any certainty. That's perhaps the reason why we should still keep referring to him as "Extrasupernatural man"—at least for a while.

The God of the Bible takes as little as ten percent that he plans to return, just like our governments do whenever they collect the little taxes from us;

we presumably see tangible results of their use either directly or indirectly. They help us with jobs that we would be reluctant to do individually or that we would sometimes never plan or think of doing for the benefit of the community. They think of elderly homes, orphanages, vulnerable and poor people, street kids, education and health services, markets, roads and whatnot. So, a lot is achieved with the little money collected from each one of us. They urge us to give while they work with "it shall be given back to you in some other ways later" vision. We lose nothing when we give, so to speak.

Where does this "Extrasupernatural man" take the whole lots of money then? No idea. What does the business owner get in return? No one knows. In case you want to stop this litany of uncertainties—"no one knows," "no clues," "no ideas"—it would be better to stop asking many questions about this man or any of his dealings.

Turning back to my fellow Africans or anyone else living on the planet where this business could be happening: If there's any physical or moral person disguising himself into this "Extrasupernatural man," I think it's better he stops such a bloody game, for peace's sake. I would implore my fellow Africans, from now on, if we have any professional actor around aspiring to win a "Hollyworld Peace Prize," he must target this man. If there's anyone around desiring to win the Nobel Peace Prize, then he must seek to nullify this man's schemes. But I should warn him to be very careful.

On the other hand, I feel sorry for the leaders who're going through such a terrible experience if they really exist. That's more than going through hell. I know they're dealing with someone who might be totally different from them, in essence—someone with either experience or wisdom that's beyond our material world and that none of us can dare to fathom. But he doesn't have any sort of compassion for inhabitants of this planet, let alone our continent. I personally wouldn't want to face such a callous man, because I would never project failure if I were to become president someday, though I've never dreamed of it even once.

Now suppose you are involved in that business, how would you feel when the eighty percent is gone? What could be your vision for running it? What would you want to achieve in doing it? Why would you involve someone who seems to be cleverer than yourself into it? I'm sorry to inform such a poor leader that he'd be a loser in that business from the day he indulges into it to the day he takes his last breath, because no country can survive on twenty percent of revenues. Anyway, I can sense what he always feels whenever that happens to him: because I know how it feels to have less. And I'm not sure he can do anything to oppose it if that is being imposed on him. I'm not sure, really.

But we should try to find some truth here. If the whole business chat is true—if it's happening around—what do our leaders then do with the remaining twenty percent? After being treacherously misled by their business partners, after having been emotionally broken down—having sworn, cursed, cried, and mourned over their unsuccessful businesses— what do they use the twenty percent for? Behind this lies the most dangerous African evil I've been talking about all through: selfishness. Most of our leaders, whether absorbed in such a dirty business or not, hardly remember us ordinary citizens. They become too self-centred: the "Me" syndrome quickly takes over and settles in. They sacrifice schools, health centers, elderly homes, roads, orphanages, factories, transport and communication facilities: they deliberately ignore all public-related services to increase their wealth. This is why I said some of our leaders are interested in nothing else but gathering wealth: We are not aware of the work the twenty percent does. Where do they keep it? For I'm sure most of us would like to know in which coffer the twenty percent is kept so we can at least remunerate some of our fellows around. Most of our leaders are so much involved in the gathering business. To quote Dr. Diescho, the executive of most of our governments continue to drift away from the people since some members of cabinets and other senior government officials are too preoccupied with their own positions and wallets instead of serving our nations. In his speech in Accra, President Obama stressed that no country can create wealth if its leaders exploit the economy to enrich themselves. Unfortunately, that's the picture of Africa since the era of independence. If the twenty percent is too little to pay teachers—as we often undermine their job even though it's what makes all of us who we are today—why can't we pay even those men in uniform?

I'm tempted to venture the best guess I can. Anyway, remember that this chapter is all about rumors, and guesses fare well in this area. And my guess is this: If it's true that eighty percent of our resources is being fraudulently taken away (which I'm still not sure about), then the remainder is also not kept in our public coffers. How would you believe that someone could become a millionaire, erect effigies at every corner of our cities in his name, and buy villas everywhere around the globe after having lost the eighty percent (from which he's supposed to get his wages) is gone? He must use the whole twenty percent to manage to do all that. And if he doesn't use the whole twenty percent, how could he become a millionaire after only a couple of days in the office?

At this point we may—if we're lucky—discover that "Extrasupernatural man" whose dealings continually shuttered us earlier: it's probably our own leaders. And if it's not them (and I also think they can't take that high risk of disguising themselves into "Extrasupernatural men"), then at least we've discovered the reason why they're involved in the 80/20 business: They're after material prosperity and self-enrichment. They accept to indulge in that business because they benefit a lot from it. They have a great deal of shares in it. They like to steal behind the names of some strange people that we can't easily face and confront. Our leaders are impostors in the true sense of the word.

The best way to help our nations is to fight that business. That's the highest level of selfishness. I believe none of us is interested in seeing millions in some individual's bank accounts. We also don't really need any villas abroad. All we need is to see our countries upgraded. And if someone were a hindrance to this journey (from Here to There), we wouldn't need him at all. He'd better do us a favor and resign. We can easily achieve our dream, especially without him around. All we need to do to reach There quickly is to get such an impostor off the road.

If there's someone among our leaders who still is unaware of our corporate dream, he better steps aside because he needs to learn some lessons. And he's lucky because he'd learn them if he so wishes. But if he's just pretending, he's not being wise enough because his pretence would indeed cause his downfall. And if he's ready to learn those lessons about our corporate dream, they're very simple but too demanding, too difficult but not impossible: "We're longing to get 'There' from 'Here,' to develop Africa"—nothing less. And so, I should say this is not time to waste whatever income one gets for his personal expenses or luxury. It's time we start moving from "Here" where we've been wasting so much time. How shameful it is to opt to be lagging behind in a world like ours that has been advancing this fast? We must seek by all means to improve the present state of affairs in our countries and advance. Enough should be enough. We must be fed up with this malevolence in Africa. We must regret the ruins we're causing and the shame we're bringing onto this potentially blessed continent, and so seek to improve in any way.

All the dictators on the continent could be addressed in the following words: "Thinking you're the peak, or you're smarter than everyone else, is a grave confusion. Thinking you're immortal is lunacy. Trying to fool your fellow countrymen is foolishness in the truest sense. Mismanaging the public treasure is a shame you could be putting on yourself and your offspring forever. Being an individualist is a deadly poison. Leading without a common vision or approval is synonymous to planning to fail. But remembering these few words is one among the keys to success."

Yet another terrifying diabolic character still is the greed of some bunch of leaders in some countries who're disturbing all the plans for development. You'd find a small group of leaders with a team of some few buddies controlling everything in the country as their private property. Many African leaders who have stepped down are always accused of this wrong: they're always accused of having misused or mismanaged their countries' resources.

For me, it seems that whoever gets power takes self-enrichment as the unique goal to achieve (no wonder they get so carried away), and if he doesn't achieve it while in the office that would be his greatest failure: for him it is an unspeakable blunder. Their priority lists seem to be starting like this: self-enrichment first, then development, if there'll be any left over.

Someone said if you want to know a person's priority just look at his expenditure, but I'd also add that if you want to know our African leaders' priorities just look at what they do. For most of them, self-enrichment seems to be essential and the rest unnecessary. And no one should comment on this utter mismanagement while they're still in the office. The order sent out to ordinary citizens by leaders seems to be: "sit down and watch us, the utterance of any word would land you into the penitentiary or something worse than that." Our leaders like to be referred to as public servants, but yet they want to be treated more like some distant royalties. If they are public servants, whom are they serving? They rule with an iron arm: absolute masters of some "kingdoms." They manage public properties as one would run his private business—without caring much about those millions of us deprived of health facilities, those going hungry to bed every night, without education, without employment . . .

To prevent this evil in the future, I would suggest the entire continent to apply the late Zambian president Levi Mwanawasa and the Liberian president Johnson Sir-Leaf's strategies toward their predecessors—Frederic Chiluba and Charles Taylor—on all the other leaders who abuse power and misuse our countries' resources. We must develop and that's one prerequisite. No leader is elected for his self-enrichment, and no one should appoint himself for the same reason either. Every leader is elected to facilitate his compatriots to get "There" from "Here"—and not to employ them for his business. We must all speak one word, and that's "development." Whoever mismanages his country's resources must be apprehended: imprisonment and confiscation of all ill-gotten properties could be the right measures to take against such a leader. Unfortunately, many of our leaders do not even have the courage to challenge their predecessors because they know very well that they are not any different.

But here is the catch: Mwanawasa and Johnson Sir-Leaf's strategies could only be applicable if they won't be accused of the same evil after they leave office. For if they'll be accused of the same wrongs then they're not setting any good example than what I call "the game of power." Because, ostensibly, many African leaders appear in disguise first—they appear first like angels to us: they'd do some good work at the beginning (probably to veil us) and then change their faces later: they ultimately show their true colors. Therefore, if their (Mwanawasa and Sir-Leaf) successors will also accuse them of mismanagement or abuse of power, then what they've been doing to their predecessors is utterly nonsensical. What I mean is, irresponsible leaders must be taken before the courts of law for their wrongs and pay back whatever they've stolen while in office, but also those who accuse them must remain above reproach. Let's stay away from 80/20 percent business if we want to develop our continent.

# Chapter Five

# The Complex Issue: Land

It's not wise to overlook the issue of land. Every one of us knows at least something about the predicament in which land has left us in Africa. It concerns each one of us, therefore, and we shouldn't ignore it. Of course, it still remains one of the most tangible assets showing and proving someone's origins in our continent and elsewhere. That's why you can still hear even today in the U.S., where some of the racial, religious or original differences are being successfully stifled. Some people are referred to Americans originally from Latin America, Africa, Europe, or Asia. Land on our continent is, in fact, a very complex issue. And today there's no sensitive issue that needs to be delicately touched like land. Who's the owner, anyway?

As far as land is concerned, one can say that history suggests that the rightful owner of a given place is the indigenous. In modern English, I think the term "indigenous" would imply somebody or something that originally or rightfully belongs to a particular place before anyone or anything else come in. In terms of people, it would mean belonging to a place before anyone else arrives there, perhaps for his discovery adventures or other climatic constraints.

And so I think it wouldn't sound strange if someone said history dictates that land in the U.S. belongs to Native Americans (also called Indians by the early explorers). That land could be said theirs because they lived there before Christopher Columbus and his team landed on the shores of America—and even long before English missionaries and other migrants moved and occupied America. In other words, before we knew America as a 'New World' it used to be an '*Old World*' to Native Americans.

Nevertheless, land ownership can be lost through either of the following ways: it is willingly given away to someone else (via any transaction), or it is snatched away, or what would be referred to as extortion in a court of law. If the rightful owner of a certain piece of land is the "indigenous"—someone who owned it before anyone else came to settle—then, historically, African land belongs to Africans. Who is an African, then? The understanding of who an African is would inhibit most of our problems related to land today. I'll try to explain this later.

According to historians still, before any colonization, Africa was inhabited by two main racial groups: White Africans, mainly found in Northern Africa in countries known as Arabic today, and black Africans living in central and southern Africa in countries known as Sub-Saharan today. In French, this is put in much clearer words: they'd say "Afrique Noire" (Black Africa) when referring to countries inhabited by a large number of people of dark skin. And "Afrique Blanche" (White Africa) refers to countries where the majority of their population has white skin—like Morocco, Tunisia, and Egypt,.

Based on this account of history, one would say that northern African land originally belongs to "White Africans," or Arabs, and central and southern African land belongs to black Africans, or "Sub-Saharans." And I believe at this point we're all being tempted to ask: In which way, then, did Africans lose their lands? I'm not sure, but I guess it's possibly through one of the above-mentioned ways: Either they willingly gave it away or it was extorted from them.

The following should be considered at this level: If they willingly gave their land to foreigners, it's foolish to claim it back. I remember in my early teenage years most of the receipts I got from shops bore these words on them: "No exchanging, no returning." This simply meant that no buyer would be allowed, in any case whatsoever, to exchange the product or item he purchased from the shop. And no purchased items would be returned after leaving the shop's premises. Even today I still don't know exactly why it was like that, but that was what one would be told to read whenever he attempted to exchange or return the purchased products for some "relevant" reasons of his own. Today I think those words would be almost similar to what we find inscribed on boards at many of our modern public playgrounds and sport facilities: "The use of these facilities is at your own risk."

And I wonder if some of us really take time to think about that inscription before they jump into the swimming pools or before they put their kids on the seesaws—they just go ahead and use them. When the thrill of enjoyment fills one's heart, it's hard to think about anything else that may interfere or repress the enjoyment. It's a pity that people wouldn't take time to think over some important things that bear so much implication on their lives like that.

To paraphrase the above for our own case, it might sound more like: "There won't be any exchange or return of land because it was done at one's own risk." And that, in essence, is not unfair.

Every transaction involving some valuable services or products seems to be always done under this principle. Every time you sign a contract or a receipt, one of you seems to be saying to the other: "You're signing it at your own risk." That's risk in the real sense: body, time, energy, money, and all. In fact, part of your life (if not all) is fully engaged—is at stake, so to speak. That's the meaning of signatures. If both parties knew beyond doubt that there'd be no problem or any clashes and if they really trusted each other, then signatures would not add anything at all, and so they wouldn't be used to seal any business. But signatures always add something to the business of a transaction. That's why we can't conclude any business without them. It seems we're aware of our own state. We know that we are so corrupt that only signatures could bind us to the promises we make and prevent us from double-crossing each other. So anyone who made the mistake of giving his land away in the past must be careful in his present and future dealings because it may cost him more than he has ever thought. He should continually bear that in mind.

Some people broke in tears before those "unmerciful" vendors, especially when they were sent by others—parents or relatives. But, unfortunately, they were always told that they should have carefully checked and approved the item before they eventually left the shop. Well, was not that the truth expressed in those words on the receipts? So, bear that in your mind, whenever it comes to land or any other valuable asset in transaction: "Don't be quick to carry out any business, for it possibly won't be returned back." And I also think this should be left so. This is true fair play.

Another example that is closer to this is gambling. I've seen owners of casinos getting enraged at people who win lots of money in their casinos. They threaten them to return the money and do all kinds of illicit things to get their money back. But there's no any right whatsoever allowing the owner of a casino to oblige the gambler to return what he has won or continue playing when he has won enough for himself and decided to leave. Returning the money won is a totally different deal—which is no longer part of the game itself—that should involve negotiation only under completely new agreements. Likewise, replaying also would involve both negotiation and persuasion. And the whole process (negotiation and persuasion) would be a success only if the beneficiary gives in or agrees— and that is, as our experience shows, not always easy or possible.

If they were forced to give it away, by any means involving threats and extortion, then they have the right to claim it and get it back. If they gave in to the threat, it must be perhaps because they were incapable to resist, or unaware of their rights, or even unaware of their land's value. But all that doesn't matter anymore.

If it wasn't their agreement to give it away, then no matter how long it has stayed in the other people's hands, it's still theirs. In addition to that, they're now aware of their rights and know their land's value—that's why they're claiming it back. I think the best way to calm this noise is either to return it back or negotiate with the rightful owner. They're the ones to decide either to allow you to continue using it or not. And this could be the solution to the matter.

In fact, what all of us should know is that there wouldn't be a nation existing somewhere without land. In order to have a nation, there should be a piece of land somewhere, and the people of that nation would only be called nationals if they were in charge of that land. It's obvious: "No land, No nation." So, if someone remembers today that somewhere back he occupied some land without the indigenous people's agreement, and if they are now claiming it back, the wisest thing he could do immediately is to either return it back or negotiate with the owner, for peace's sake. If he reacts to this in some different way, it may rouse either a cold war or an armed conflict. And this is the threshold we're standing at. We must try to apply some of these ideas in order to avoid unending conflicts on the continent. I don't think there would be any joy in keeping what does not belong to you when the owner earnestly wants it back.

Nonetheless, the great challenge remains to know who sold this land (if it was sold at all). Who took the responsibility of the entire land and decided to share or sell it without consulting others? The fact that we're still struggling with settling this matter on the continent is clear proof that probably the dealer didn't consult everyone else before he sold it. That, in our world, should have been the highest form of egomania. It also clearly shows that perhaps it was not his private property, and so he had no right to share or sell it. For whose benefit did he sell it? Who supported his decision? It certainly seems that no indigenous got involved in this business. Then who caused this? If any one of us knows this man, he should confront him because he might be standing with an ultimate and durable solution to this problem. He might have imagined or planned beforehand how to help each one of his fellow landless countrymen when this issue gets serious some other time like today. This man can, beyond any doubt, help us calm this problem easily.

Moreover, and this is unbearable to many, most of us feel it's still unfair to have suffered oppression and exploitation before independence, and then have no right to our own land after achieving independence. In fact, most of us never stop asking themselves how a landless man could be independent. No wonder why most of us get so easily enraged when talking about land. On the other hand, I believe it would be fair to say that any foreign settler who acquired his land from indigenous people, via any transaction whatever—it shouldn't matter whether he is African, Asian, European, American or Australian—the land should be his. All he may be courteously asked to do at this level is to effectively use the land by making it productive. He also should be regularly reminded that he's still liable to any business agreement he signed with the owner during the deal.

And if there's someone who bought or occupied enough land while others were still not interested in working the land or away in exile, or poor, or even denied any right to acquire land by some colonial regimes, it would be better to apply the principle that anyone with two cloaks should give one to his fellow who has nothing—which means that anyone with much must try to share. This is true negotiation and reconciliation.

But what we often fail to understand is that today an African is no longer defined by his skin color, his beliefs, his language, or his culture. The word "African" has transcended all that. In fact, today you wouldn't easily know who is African or not. And this puts all of us in the same position. Grabbing the land from one fellow in order to give it to another would be setting up an unending fire, because if acquiring land is based on being African then none of us is undeserving. That's why only negotiation can help us settle this matter. And in negotiation there's always one party that is advantageous, and the success of the whole process depends on him. He has the final say, so to speak. Let's hope that people would be convinced to share some of their lands during such negotiations. We must therefore keep our hope alive. That's what I promised to explain.

Finally, here's the most important thing to grasp: Land is meaningless if it's unproductive." There's no point in claiming a piece of land you don't intend to use. "To just have land won't benefit you anything if you can't get anything from it." More plainly, if you can't produce tomatoes from the land you're claiming, why would you prevent someone else from producing them? The wisest thing to do in all this would be to allow other fellow countrymen (regardless of their origin) with potential use the land and make it productive for the entire community's benefit—to stop hunger from hitting our continent, so to speak. And that's the beginning of our true freedom and development.

# Chapter Six

# What Do We Do With Our Land?

In the previous chapter I dealt with an issue I acknowledged to be complex. Of course, the land issue is very thorny in Africa today. Some of our fellow brothers lost their land during colonial time; that's why they're still claiming it back. A question could be asked right here: Are they claiming it back with the intention to make it productive, or to simply own land? Both can be true. There's yet another question for clarification: Should they be encouraged to continue claiming it back?

Before we answer this question, we should first try to ignore those who don't have land now and look at those who have it. In some of our countries land is in the hands of citizens "rightful owners" from the day they marked independence. And so, it's not as difficult for a citizen to acquire land as in other countries. These are the countries we should first look at. And, looking at them, it seems that the only thing we can't manage properly or invest in is land. I'm aware that I'll collect some objections here. Well, this is said based on my experience and direct observation. And I'm warning you as I did before, if you get nothing from this, you'd better read another chapter.

I never stop wondering why people should die of starvation in Ethiopia bordering some lands where food could be produced. I never understand why such a fertile country like the DRC should import a huge amount of food from its neighboring countries and even from South Africa. It's inconceivable to see countries with some arable lands begging for thousands of tons of food from the World Food Programme.

Some time back, I used to defend those countries by saying that they don't have appropriate tools to work their land—but this defense caught me in a trap. The trap was that if we can't easily get funds to buy agricultural machinery, then it may be almost impossible to maintain mining companies. But these mining companies are always functioning and they rarely go bankrupt. This is enough proof that they're in good hands. If we don't have enough funds to buy irrigation and watering equipments and tractors, where do we get sufficient funds to set up these mining companies and maintain them? This is where I always got confused.

After all this, I would quickly conclude that we don't have heart for our land as we do for mines. This gives the impression of being true anyway.

I still remember back in my village, a fisherman was more highly respected than a crop farmer—not because one job could make you dirtier or smellier than the other, but simply because, probably, one job could get you quicker cash than the other. Unfortunately, that misperception persists up to now. Farming, for many chaps of my color, is considered to be a detestable job reserved only for some folks willing to connect with dirt. Yet and this would sound quite shocking to most of us—dirt seems to be the most productive thing. This is really a matter of experience.

So, those engaged in illegal mining or fishing business in DRC, Angola, Liberia, and other countries would therefore be elevated to higher classes. And this makes people run from farming to fishing, and especially to illegal mining and other businesses. But I firmly believe the opposite is worth doing. I'm not saying that everybody should abandon mining and fishing for farming; all I'm trying to say is that all must be balanced.

I said somewhere that I was always drawing a quick conclusion that we have no heart for land. Yes, it's true that is a quick conclusion. To say that we all don't have heart for our land is trying to run faster than a bullet because not everyone on the continent is lazy. And this brings us back to the group we previously ignored for a while: those who are desperately waiting for the restitution of their lands. I suggested that they should be ignored for a while—and, of course, for a specific reason—but I guess not everyone liked my suggestion then. I'll explain my reason.

Let's now attempt to suggest an answer to the question we left earlier: "Are they claiming their land back with the intention to make it productive, or to simply own it?" This question would ultimately bring us in front of the following hypotheses.

They might be claiming their land back for what I would call good intentions—to work it. This group that I call "Second" (because they came after the first group that took full control of their land immediately after independence), is greatly privileged because in life we believe "we learn from mistakes and failures" either made by others or ourselves. What I mean by this is that the "Second" group has seen the "First" group. This group failed to make its land productive though we all thought they could have some potential to produce at least some crops. The second group is lucky because it has learned a lot from the first group's failure. I believe they're coming out in full speed, so they would do something that was never achieved.

They want to prove their ability and potential to the rest of the continent. They're eager to achieve something tangible despite their late emergence. That's the only motive behind their noise, I guess. They'd never stop claiming their land back because they're totally convinced once they get onto it, starvation would remain a word without any meaning in Ethiopia and the rest of the continent. For that reason, I would advise those land distributors (whoever they are) to give these folks the chance to fulfill their long-awaited dream.

My advice to these fellows (if they can listen to me at all) is that they shouldn't blame the "First" group for failing to make their land productive. As C.S. Lewis would say, those in the "Second" group were like someone patiently waiting outside behind many rooms, trying to figure out which of the various doors in the big hall is the right one to knock at. When he happens to knock and enter the right door, he realizes that the long wait has done him some kind of good, which he wouldn't have had otherwise. So, their delay and waiting has helped them to observe and clearly see what should be the next right step to make. Their success is being made clear through the "First" group's failure; otherwise they would all fail. Think of the continent's fate if that could happen.

There's also another possibility we should never overlook: they may also fail just like the "First" group. But if they fail, then they're the worst of all. I guess at this point some readers are already expressing some kind of annoyance. They've had enough of my negative thoughts that they can't bear any more. Maybe they're already complaining that all I can do is look at things from a negative angle, or consider Africans as a bunch of incompetents. That's not it! I'm sorry to those who are feeling like that on this point, but I'm in the quest of making some points clear "Here" so we won't stumble or fall again in our journey to 'There"—that's the aim of this book, which I consider a guide to anyone willing to move ahead.

So, it's possible that those from the "Second" group may also fail to do what the "First" group failed to. They may get their land back, but have no crops produced from it. They may finally get their land back after having identified all the reasons behind the 'First' group's failure. They may fail even after they had enough time to evaluate, analyze and remove all possible constraints behind each of those reasons.

But success should be obvious to members of this group. Could their failure be because of lack of appropriate means to work their land, too? If the answer to this question is yes, then I have to admit that we've settled on a wrong planet; maybe Jupiter is our planet. Let's hope all will go better once we step on Jupiter than it is for us here on Earth now. It's bad news but, and I'm afraid, somehow it seems we won't make it here. And I'm not sure if I know why.

But if the answer is no, then we have to leave behind all the hearsay chat and try to think of another possible factor contributing to this: laziness. But it's also quasi-nonsensical to evoke the question of laziness on a continent where at least a number of villages manage to feed their townships by using some rudimentary tools for crop farming. One possible question I may be asked here would be whether such people are also lazy or not. I also think they're not. All they need are modern tools and some information and training to improve their work for a better and abundant harvest.

Before I move on, I would like to indicate something at this stage: If these brave villagers do work the land in order to prevent *only* their own families from starvation, if they're producing their products to *only* feed this limited number of people (as small as their families), or if they're *only* selling their products to cover their families' basic needs, then they're still far from what I mean by working the land. Remember, earlier on I said that we want to see our food stores full every day, in every season. Then this automatically implies that unless they make our warehouses full, they'd never do what I mean yet what the continent needs: plenty of food, breaking the walls of our warehouses and overflowing to Addis Ababa and Darfur.

At this moment, I can see how impossible it is for villagers to fill up our warehouses despite their earnest courage, because our warehouses cannot be made full with rudimentary tools. Whoever wants to fill them needs modern machinery for farming—machinery they don't possess. Therefore our governments (or whoever's in charge) should provide modern machinery to these men who have shown their courage to fill our food stores. They've proven that they're the only people who can produce enough food even "There." They must be trusted, trained and equipped for that task.

I commend these villagers because they contribute enormously to many people's lives in most of our towns. I wish all of them could get some space in those special graveyards reserved for heroes and heroines because they're deserving. As you could see, and if you can believe it, they're more than those so-called "freedom fighters" who fought for the liberation of our countries from foreign oppression, and for whom those graveyards are often reserved. The reason is: who knows if oppressors could have come back to their senses and allow us to live as independent as they were? Anyway, the essence of those struggles itself was based on that hope. Hope that "oppressors" would consider letting us off. There was that possibility because there were two ultimate options: either oppression goes on, or it stops. One or the other could have prevailed. But if these devoted villagers in some countries stop working their land or reduce the quantity of their production, there'd be only one result: deaths will be recorded in most of our townships and their outskirts.

These men free us from starvation, they energize us for labor in our factories, mining companies, and fishing businesses. It was sung somewhere in Africa that: "In order to work, one needs to eat." Is not this much the same as saying, "Without strong and courageous villagers there'd be no harvest, and without harvest there'd be no food, and without food none of us would go to work?" That song should have been a praise hymn dedicated to those villagers. We must hail these men and shout: "Long live heroes and heroines!" We must wish them long lives because their early deaths would cause thousands or even millions of early departures. You may be asking now, "What is the importance of the heroes' story in here?" I will tell you why: These folks often go unnoticed despite all the efforts they make—of course not behind the scenes. It's being ungrateful if we disregard their contribution to most of our countries. When I call them heroes, I mean it.

Remember somewhere in this chapter I raised the issue of laziness? I don't have much to say about this, but perhaps I'm one of those lazy folks who would not easily accept to touch the soil. All I can tell anyone in my position is that he must change his attitude towards land. Land itself and even working it is not something for dirty boys. I love that washing powder advert: "Dirt is good." Yes, dirt is absolutely good, especially in agriculture. We must work our land if we want to venture into any other business. And even for any other work, no matter how tiring it might be, one has to keep the right attitude.

In a workaholic world like ours, I think it would be fair to advise one to stop being a spectator and encourage him to be involved in the system because all seems to be coming from our busyness. Therefore, we must stop sleeping on duty, wandering, and messing around. We must stop waiting for the manna; it ceased to fall thousands of years ago. We must avoid showmanship and pride; they're only good at causing one's downfall. We must stop being obsessed with our clothes and skins; they can't make us anything without food. We must always remember that ultimate joy comes from work. The only secret to enjoy your job is to love it, no matter what kind of work. Only that reduces stresses at the end of the day. Maybe that's what we should apply when it comes to agriculture. Research show that what makes us tired, robs us of our joy and stresses us is not overwork but doing the job you don't like. So, everyone should love his job and work it: that's the beginning of our development. We must never be fooled by the reality portrayed by the media.

We must stop dreaming to live the reality of magazines and televisions if we hate work. About ninety-five percent of men and women we view every day in our movies and magazines are all working. They don't just fill up streets, sit, parade and talk to exhibit some "happy-clappy" clips to make us feel good. Anyway, making us happy is even one of their duties. We must stop lazing around. We must get off streets and engage into something productive we can initiate. We must always remember that we have only two main job creators: The government and ourselves (self-employment). We shouldn't throw it all to our governments, because we're also accountable.

It's prudent to know beforehand that it's difficult to get employed if you're lazy; yet, on the other hand, it's very easy for someone to discover that he can't work hard. By this I mean that any job you get must find you hardworking, it shouldn't make you one. If our hope is that we will only get off streets and learn to work hard until some imaginary day when our governments offer us employments, it may be a hopeless anticipation. We may suffer terribly to acquaint ourselves with the rhythm of the jobs we get because we were not so used to working hard. My emphasis is that we must try to find something that keeps us busy even now, before our governments meet our needs.

They might be claiming the land for what I call: Bad intention or "waste," to have the land simply for the sake of owning it. It's naïve to claim the land back for the sake of just getting it. I'm quite aware that now I'm going to walk this path alone. Not many people will really compliment me for what I'd like to prove from this. I guess my job in this book should be to state some facts. Anyway, I think I should concentrate on those who're lending me their ears at least for a short time.

One of my friends, a fellow countryman at university, once told me that it doesn't matter whether the land is used or not. What matters is to get it back first because it's ours—it's for Africans. I believe he was still holding on the old definition of who an African is. I'm convinced when he said we must get the land back he was referring to the people of dark skin. And this today is so misleading because, as I said in the previous chapter, the term African implies a lot more than that today.

We must get the land back because it's ours! This seems to be the only argument available on the market and the one most spoken among my peers today. In fact it has been difficult from time to time for me to disagree because this sounds logical to many. Now I think I must also put my opinion readily available in this book. What matters to me now is only to make my opinion open to everybody but what anyone does with it is another question.

First of all, I firmly believe that nothing on Earth exists for the sake of just being there. Nothing exists as result of some mishap. There's always a purpose attached to everything around. In that way nothing is purposeless, let alone our land. Therefore, the first thing one should do when he gets any portion of land is to make it productive. That is its purpose, I believe.

Secondly, everyone should always keep in mind that whoever gives him something is delighted in his using it. If he doesn't, the giver feels he should have given it to someone else who would use it effectively. A teacher who hands out workbooks to his learners, for example, expects each one to use them. Whoever refuses to use them is a rebel, so to speak. And the feeling or the reaction of the teacher would be to get the books back, because it doesn't make any sense to hold them and not use them for the purpose for which they were handed out. I'm talking out of experience! Thirdly, the next person, call him neighbor if you want, out of envy, feels he should grab it from you if you can't use it when he thinks he can or he needs it. He feels he must put an end to this appalling waste. I guess that this may be one of the reasons why foreign settlers occupied our land.

So, those who think one should get the land for the sake of just owning it because it's rightfully theirs are, in my opinion, missing the point. That would never help Africa to develop. We must always remember the "First" group that failed to use their land and caused terrible hunger in their countries and on the continent at large. Now the "Second" group should claim their land back for one objective only: good intention. Work the land and make it productive. They must not keep their land unproductive. If they keep it unproductive, they'd make it purposeless, and naturally land is not a purposeless asset. They'd also discourage the giver or the distributor who may grab it from them anytime because of their failure to manage it properly: the failure to unleash its full potential. Moreover, they'd stir up envy in their neighbors who may be tempted to grab it from them as a result of their mismanagement. And so the situation would be more hopeless, especially in our own case. We should therefore check the motives behind our claims to get land back. I personally would never claim any land I don't intend to use because I know it will become useless if it's unproductive. Should it be kept unproductive? This is a question that begs for everyone's wisdom, because its answer determines the entire continent's fate.

# Chapter Seven

# **When?**

I suspect that, in the last chapter, I uttered something that made some of you question my skin color. Maybe at this stage some of you would like to know who I am, exactly, and what kind of people I'm referring to, from which continent I'm compiling the chapters of this book and which side I'm backing up. Well, if that is anyone's concern, I'll try to be as honest as I can. I'm not interested in whether someone is legally or illegally occupying land, or illegally or legally claiming it back. It's none of my business anyway.

However, the only side I'm backing up is of those who are making (or will continually make) our food stores full. My point is that we need food to make the first step from "Here" to "There." In order to make even the smallest move, one needs an appropriate energizer to fill his stomach. And so, if there's anyone occupying a piece of land failing to produce enough food even for few houses in his suburb, he has parted company with me.

But anyone who doesn't have land now, or has it and never plans to work, or who feels he can't make it productive for his community's benefit when he gets it, he's not with me too. Remember, land becomes useless when it's not productive. If you know you can't afford to cover all expenses required to produce enough tomatoes for a few people in your suburb, you better give the chance to someone else who can do it. I mean instead of enjoying looking at your fellows cooking their food without tomatoes while you're occupying the land that could help them get tomatoes, step aside and allow someone else with more potential to produce them.

Now some people may think that I'm so worried about the shortage of tomatoes in my country or on the continent. They might also think that I grew up in a place where a tomato is a favorite or a scarce fruit, but the opposite is very true. My using tomatoes here as an illustration is simply to help each one of us understand that at least fruits such as tomatoes should be produced everywhere on the continent. Tomatoes and other fruits should not be imported at all. Wherever one sees tomatoes in these chapters, he can substitute them with any other kind of basic food in his village—a cassava, an apple, or a potato for example. Before I move on, I would like to clarify something I've been repeatedly saying. Up to this level, you may have noticed that I've been talking about food production whenever I mentioned land. Of course my emphasis is on agriculture (farming), as I know that is the primary utility of land everywhere.

I don't remember having seen or heard anyone in Africa allowed to dig minerals he discovers on his farm. My observation is that one is allowed to occupy a piece of land where he's expected to settle or use to produce only agricultural-related products. That's the reason why I've been talking more about producing tomatoes or maize instead of gold, silver, or diamond. I'm well aware that land is a multi-service asset. It involves everything on it and in it. Therefore, if what makes the land issue complex in Africa is that minerals have to be exploited among other things on the farms, that automatically sets it beyond what I'm able to deal with. In clear words, I mean if those "illegally" occupying land now and those "legally" claiming it back are to dig minerals on their farms, I would suggest that none of them should be allowed to settle on them. If anyone expects more than that from this book, then these chapters are only going to leave him clueless.

Now, the one thing that I think made some people question my nationality and perhaps my skin color could be the statement I made in the previous chapter: "It seems to me that the only thing we can't manage or invest in is the land." I tried to explain why I made this statement in the same chapter and the rest of the defense is what I'm going to give in this one. The title of this chapter is a question: When? This is showing how uncertain I still am about some things and would like to know when we are going to properly manage our land and when we are going to start investing in it. I'd rather remain static in my view: We have to admit that we are still unable to manage or invest in the land.

One tangible example I can give to support my argument is that of farmers who left Zimbabwe and only after few days were given land in Nigeria, the most overpopulated nation in Africa. I never expected that an overpopulated country with the most educated population on the continent would give land to any foreigner to settle and use. Why wouldn't Nigeria give that land to some of their millions of landless citizens? I don't know, but I can only guess: Perhaps no Nigerian could afford to use land effectively. Say my guess is correct, then Nigerian leaders were afraid that they would not maximize their land's potential if they give it to someone who would only waste it, making it unproductive. For them it was better to sell it to foreigners. That's the right decision, but all the parties involved in buying and selling or whatever deal it is, should always remember that they're liable to every business agreement they sign. This would prevent any danger in the long run.

If Nigeria decided to give its land to foreigners in order to produce enough food at last, it's excellent. I believe the leaders thought: "Why should we cook our relish without tomatoes while there are people around who can produce them for the entire community?" I say it's excellent because it's everything I mean in this book. But if Nigeria gave its land to foreigners because no Nigerian could in fact work it, then there is a serious problem. And now, at least, one can clearly understand why I said a moment ago that we have to admit that we are still unable to manage or invest in our land. When, then, are we going to learn to invest in our land?

If our problem is lack of financial resources, then we should adopt the Nigerian way. But if our problem is laziness or some inability to manage land, then the entire African leadership needs a thorough review. But here is the catch: in case we adopt the Nigerian way then the land issue would ever remain complex and impossible to solve because those who don't have it now may probably not get it forever. To put this in simple words, unless there're no Nigerians in need of land, this should not be seen as a problem at all. But if there are many Nigerians who need land who are being ignored by a government that attends more quickly to foreigners than its own citizens, surrendering could be the wisest response from the landless. On the other hand, if we decide not to adopt the Nigerian way, then that self-confidence says a lot. It shows our readiness and willingness to invest more in agriculture. This means that we're willing to improve our budgets and get to work. That's exactly what I mean when I talk about land in these chapters. But whichever road we take, two options are inevitable in the end:

1) *The Nigerian way.* This is a belief that Africa still needs to gather enough resources before it indulges into land business. We still need more time to persuade one another to work, but in the meantime (during the time of collection of resources and persuasion) we need something to help us make things happen. Instead of keeping the land unproductive till some imaginary time in the far future when all the requirements would be met, it is better to allow someone else (regardless of his nationality or origin) use it in the meantime. For Nigeria, production is what counts, nothing else.

2) *The Mugabe conviction.* This implies that we can now get rid of all foreigners from our land, meaning that we are ready to manage and invest in our own land. Our resources alone are capable of covering all expenses required. We are no longer incapable. We have gone through a long learning process enough to provide us with all necessary skills required for the work. Though we could be unable to manage it, the fact of having it would encourage and make us strong while, and I guess, applying "trial and error" lest we lose it forever to foreigners out of fear, an inferiority complex or low self-esteem. "You'd never become a blacksmith if you don't take risk with metals," so to speak. I believe that's the idea behind Mugabe's attitude.

Now maybe some readers want to know which of the two formulas is the best to employ. Well, my answer to that is: neither of them is good or bad. Remember, I've been stressing that we can never get "There" from "Here" with our empty stomachs. So, no matter how strong we may pretend to be, only food can boost us for any other business. Therefore both can be bad if they don't provide enough food, whereas both can work if they make our food stores full.

However, here is the quick overview of the two ultimate options: If the Nigerian way is just a waiting process (an invented strategy to allow Nigerians meet all the requirements: money and courage to work their land), then it still gives hope to landless citizens. But if that's how land issue will *always* be handled in Nigeria, then there's nothing to hope for.

Surrendering and forgetting, as I said earlier, would be the wisest response from the landless.

The waiting process would allow every other landless citizen to meet all the necessary requirements by learning from those foreigners who are currently working that land.

The Mugabe conviction, on the other hand, can only be beneficial if what he believes is true. If we can now work and invest in our land by covering every single expense from our own resources, then it is my dream, too. But if it is just an assumption (and we have seen it in his own country) or a wishful thinking that Africans can do it when they really cannot, then I'm afraid of people dying of hunger all over the continent.

I first used the example of Nigeria giving its land to foreigners as a proof of our inability to manage or invest in our land. The second and last example is of hundreds of young graduates from our colleges and universities. Every year there are hundreds of our youth graduating in agriculture. Where do they go? What are they currently doing? Why is it that the more their number increases, the more famine strikes our continent? It seems that these guys are joining other businesses after they receive their degrees. If that is true, can that be due to lack of support from our governments? And if our governments are unable to support these guys, why do they still allow that course in our colleges and universities? If these folks cannot be supported, what other strategies do our governments develop to eradicate hunger on the continent?

I think it's a waste of both money and time trying to train people in a field they would not practice later. It's not wise to train people in agriculture only to see them turn into soccer stars, models, and artists later. Well, it can only be successful if letting a stick in water eventually turns it into an aquatic creature. But if by its very nature a stick is not an aquatic creature, then leaving it in the waters for centuries is no different from trying to turn black into white.

If our governments are incapable of employing these guys after obtaining their degrees, then I think it would be better to cancel the course, too. If that knowledge would not be used at all—and if Africa would not benefit anything from that course—it is better to stop it altogether. Remember everything becomes useless if it's not used. I mean our governments should not make us believe a lie that some imaginary day these guys are going to be useful by only training them or maintaining the course in our colleges and universities whereas the reality is nothing else but a perpetual lie. Our governments ought to support these people at any cost if they mean to eradicate hunger on the continent.

Also to the young graduates, if they're taking that course just for the sake of getting their degrees and then join other businesses later, they're not giving any chance to themselves, let alone our crumbling continent. They're not wise enough. In this way they're suppressing our continent's progress. The endeavor to get "There" doesn't seem to be a priority to them at all. It seems that the development of Africa is not their dream. How could they respond to the vision of hunger eradication? And how do they expect the continent develop if our land remains unproductive? Their response to these questions determines the entire continent's fate. The way they visualize the future of this continent would reveal their involvement in its development. Their need to see Africa developed determines how interested, fast, slow or compromising they would be in the whole process.

On the other hand, why are our governments unable to support these guys? It seems that our governments do not trust these young graduates. And, as I have observed, this is another mistake our governments make: instead of giving a piece of land to a young man, they would rather give it to an old man (usually a freedom fighter comrade) who may only use it for few years before he dies. I wonder why they shouldn't entrust land to some of these young graduates, then appoint some technical advisors (wise old men)—regardless of their origin—for them. I'm not saying this to advocate for people of my age, but my whole imagination is now wrapped around young and vigorous men—surrounded by experienced and skilled old men—who would possibly keep the land productive for many years. I have nothing to do with age groups. It's not the conflict of generations either; we can cut all that out. All I want to see is the land producing food consistently.

My summary of this chapter points out some reason why I think both the governors and the governed are so reluctant to manage or invest in the land. In my view, we are simply not willing to work our land. My observation is this: we are naturally impatient, always driven by haste. Whenever we do something we expect quick results. This is what I call "microwave magic" attitude. That's why you'll find most of us going for expensive German cars now while sparing nothing for our children's future. We would rather buy the most expensive clothes to wear for one occasion at the expense of our homes. We make so many useless, exorbitant expenses for some short ecstasy and ignore so many important life investments. We are a people with a vision that does not go beyond where our eyes see. We are a "now" addicted race, I would say. Unfortunately, we miss the point when we think that way because, except in magic, everything else takes time.

To make my summary short, I mean we're more comfortable with fishing for instance, because it would probably not take us thirty minutes before we catch a fish than it is to eat a ripe mango from a tree planted at the same time we went fishing. The revenue from fishing business would be quicker, even daily than it could be when one wants money from selling oranges. So, the time spent in the business, not the cost involved, remains the scary issue for most of us.

The same applies to our governments. I think they're the worst. They're more comfortable with investing in the exploitation of diamonds than in maize production. Because, probably getting a diamond would not take them months and the smallest of it could buy all the maize produced in an entire harvest season. Therefore, they think it's far better to go for diamond business (and get quick cash) because it may likely breed maize indirectly. Sadly, the same quick cash is spent on quick services. For them, the maize business would only delay the cash flow or only get them a few coins in the end. In many African countries, thanks to the alarming rate of corruption, there are two newly appointed ministers: one for agriculture and another for finances, economy or mines. The latter is expected to become richer than the former—in people's minds—before they even pick up their pens or boost their computers to resume work. Any country overwhelmed by this sort of perception is encountering terrible starvation in the long run, no matter how fertile its land may be. DRC is one typical example.

One thing I want to mention before I close this chapter is that, comparing farming and digging gold (agriculture and mining) is a fatal mistake. Economically, they're not of the same value. I can plainly declare that precious stones are more expensive than apples and bananas. Here I'm trying to determine the value of an item by its cost. Yet I know that the cost of an item can only make it costly but not necessarily important. The importance of an item is, according to my understanding, determined by its impact on someone's life. What is the impact of precious stones on our bodies compared to that of food? Is there really any other purpose for precious stones if not only ornamental? Yet many of us don't even know the word ornament itself. That would show the importance of those two things. In many cases, people who are driven by value in making their choices are the ones who often make queerest mistakes.

It may happen by mistake that someone asserts that an airplane is more valuable than the breath of life. This is a terrible mistake that may be caused by asking yet another wrong question like: "How much does each one of them cost?" Of course, on the surface the answer would be: "Zero coin, for breath but millions for an aircraft." The price of an aircraft, in this case, may make it expensive but not necessarily important: the breath in our nostrils is important than the largest jet.

Likewise, producing tomatoes is more important than concentrating on digging gold and copper. The truth is, everyone (including mine dealers) needs food to survive but not everybody needs gold. This means that you can go on living your life (if you have food) without bothering much about even knowing the color of gold.

Our governments must take this to heart: there are people all over their countries who don't care about even knowing how bright, transparent or costly a diamond is, but every one of them needs food. So, they must not sacrifice every single resource of the country for mining business only. Not all of them need it. I'm not saying that we should forget about mining and sustain agriculture only. What I mean is that if you know that food is number one in people's lives, then it's better to also spend considerable resources in producing enough of it. Let's spend according to our needs' priorities. What comes first on the list should get more and so on.

I believe now some of you would like to know something about those nations that do not have minerals how they squander their little resources too. I also wonder why agriculture should not be their priority in this case, but what I know is that every country is driven by something lucrative that makes it sacrifice agriculture. Whatever that may be, my aim for writing this is to help our leaders shift. I'm completely convinced that many countries can successfully eradicate hunger if our leaders stop focusing and spending more on diamonds, gold, and copper. Of course agriculture takes time but its impact is of continual positive effects on human lives.

# Chapter Eight

# Religious Wars in Africa

Most of us have already heard about "Holy Wars." Sometimes it sounds funny but more unpleasant. But we need to tackle it because that, too, stands as a stumbling block to our continent's development. If people cannot cooperate or cohabit because of religion, they can hardly agree on anything else. What you know as a "Holy War" in the Middle East is what I'm calling a "Religious War" in this section. It is not easy to deal with this issue, but I'll try. I feel it's difficult to address this issue on a continent full of theists, atheists, and agnostics.

Theists believe God exists. I'm one of them but I also believe we shouldn't wage any war in order to draw people closer to our God. I'll explain it later. Atheists believe there's no God and that people only form their own idea of God in their attempt to explain the unexplainable. According to them, the whole idea of a supreme power behind everything is simply a human invention. Since they believe there's no God, I think the question of religious or holy wars would not make any sense to them at all. Agnostics say they can't know because nothing about God can be known with any certainty. So, I guess, for them, too, the holy war is a story to stop at once.

I'm a monotheist who believes that nobody should engage into any type of war to draw people to God via his religion. I know about countries where Buddhists, Hindus, and a handful of Christians coexist peacefully.

There are countries where polytheists and monotheists live without serious confrontations. I remember a country where Judaism and Christianity raise no big problems at all. But I hardly remember a country where Islam and Christianity live without confronting each other. These countries are either in an armed conflict (the example of Nigeria, Sudan, and others) or in a cold war (like in Tanzania, Burundi, Zanzibar, and other countries). Whether these two religions are monotheistic or polytheistic (but both of them claim to be monotheistic), I believe atheists and agnostics are busy studying how different their gods are. It means that the thing they have been denying the most is being revealed to them clue by clue through the actions of practicing Christians and Muslims. Our claims and practices in the name of our gods is a firsthand portrayal of how our gods really are. Here is where our wisdom is put to the test, because we would be the most preposterous impostors in human history if our claims in the name of our gods appear to be simply our ruthlessness toward fellow human beings. And, to put it in the words of President Obama, defining oneself in opposition to someone who worships a different prophet, has no place in the twenty-first century. We are all God's children.

These gods are very strange gods: They don't acknowledge each other. One is totally evil before the other. Each of them wants to prove how good he is and constantly tries to show how evil is the other. One of them appears to be so patient with those who do not respond to his call and yet the other is so intolerant. He can't tolerate anyone going his own way or joining the other god. He orders his followers to get, at any cost, everyone to respond to his call. Anybody who continues to harden his heart or continues to rebel against him is to be put to death. The other god's brain seems to be addled by love, and so he simply says: "It doesn't matter who responds to my call. Besides, they're free to do what they want, but I'll wait until they listen." He allows every human being to exercise his free will and choose between coming back to him or continuing his way or even joining the other god. So each god seems to be making propaganda to plunder the other god's camp to populate his, to get everybody to his side.

And this may turn out to be a disaster to some in the long run because only the "good" god would get some good gifts to reward his followers and the bad god wouldn't be able to produce or deliver anything good. Bad is always doomed to breed bad. This shows that life's choices are not mere milk and water, as it is often caricatured by some of us at the moment. Good choices now are likely to get one good gifts, both now and in future. It's not my intention to criticize any of those two religions but, from what we see through their followers' actions, I think that's how their gods operate.

Yet above all else, I'm always stunned by this: Despite all those glaring divergences and contrasts, Christians and Muslims meet somewhere. They all share one crucial point of view: Judgment. They all believe that whether you respond to their gods' call or not, you'll find yourself before the Judgment Seat some day. And on that day, there'll be no more choice to whether accept their gods' call or not, because the "free will" faculty shall be made ineffective. It will be the time when everyone will have to bear the consequences of his response to the call: whether he chose to say yes to that call and went back or he said no, then recklessly continued his way or joined the other god. Don't take this as a sermon; it's not my intention to deliver one. But there *is* something I want to say.

If their gods have set some day for judgment ahead of everyone's life, then they must be some sort of "liberal" gods who let every one of us run himself freely (not like an automaton or a puppet) in the present time. But the consequences of every choice we make now will have an endless effect on our lives afterward. And if these gods operate with such a broad idea of human freedom in their minds, I don't think they would urge their followers to wage any war to bring them everyone back. But if they don't acknowledge to have let anyone use his free will now, then I don't even know why they should set any day for judgment where punishment seems to be based on choices made during someone's lifetime. Judgement Day is irrational in a world without free will. And in a world devoid of free will, nobody could compromise with the rules that are set. The absence of free will means coercion toward anything available. In such a world, nobody would dodge because no any other option is offered, and so everyone would be bound to conformity. Unfortunately, that does not give any picture of the world we live in. Our own experience shows that we're made to live freely and make free choices. Naturally, human beings are not living like automatons; they're free beings surrounded by choices all around, even the simplest choices like what to eat on a particular day and at what time. I believe that is the reason why these gods have set the judgment day ahead because they are prepared to punish whoever ignores their call now. It's the day that justice shall finally be offered though seemingly delayed, so to speak.

Having left such freedom of choice to mankind, I believe attempting to win everyone's souls to these gods is not what they would expect from their followers. I'm inclined to think that this free will is the thing that will get some souls closer to these gods eternally (if it makes wise choices) but it is also the thing that will prevent others from enjoying their eternity together with these gods (if it makes bad choices).

We should also know that having free will does not guarantee one to make good choices. But I guess that any good god would always wish the best to everyone caught in the predicament of making choices. By this I mean he wants them to make some good and wise choices that would lead to eternal enjoyment. Therefore these gods would instruct their followers to always leave room for choice—the choice to either accept or refuse—to whoever they want to win for them. They would not pull them about and manipulate them like some toys to follow wherever they lead them as they pull the strings. Such a relationship cannot be enjoyable at all. That's what I promised to explain.

The issue of religion is all about worship. I feel that, to some extent, there's no need for us to even include the issue of "freedom of religion" in our constitutions. But then I've realized that everything about our social behavior—or what we call "morality"—stipulated in our constitutions is not really new stuff. They were all inside us long before they made part of what we now call "constitutions," and so is the issue of worship. And for that reason, it must be included in our constitutions for emphasis.

Men only copied what was already written on the inside: our hearts. That's why the issue of religion being included in our countries' constitutions is no different from the law that forbids murder: because we have something already whispering to us that we shouldn't take out someone's life. And that's why it appears so disgusting to all of us when it happens. Then what we read on the papers of our constitutions is similar to what we hear from our consciences. Their appearance on papers is nothing else but an emphasis showing how important these things are to us. And for that reason, the "freedom of religion" must appear on every constitution of all our countries and it must be enforced, especially when it comes to its implementation.

At this point I suspect that someone is tempted to ask why it should be enforced. The freedom of religion must be enforced because worship is something that is done freely. You don't force people to worship God. That would be a pretentious act of worship and, in essence, no serious God would accept any pretense. We must also understand that men everywhere have a strong impulse urging them to worship even if they disagree on whom or what to worship.

People all over our continent (because of that permanent need for worship), worshiped long before they knew anything about Christianity, Islam, Hinduism, Buddhism, Judaism, and the rest. Still, because of this need for reverence, some people worshiped things in nature: sun, moon, animals, trees, rivers, fire, etc. Some even made their own people their objects for worship. Then because of the uncertainty of whom or what to worship, people fell in prostrate before anything they favored, held dear, or respected. And still more, because of this disagreement, even people from one country or one region, the same hamlet or town, same tribe or clan found themselves splitting into different camps when it came to worship. They would go before two totally different objects and kneel in worship, expecting all of them to have the same power or, if not equal in power, at least all of them could do them some good. That's why we are still split into three main groups I mentioned earlier in this chapter: theists, atheists and agnostics. And again theists are also divided into two big groups: monotheists and polytheists. I don't know much about atheists and agnostics, but I believe, based on what we're experiencing in our camp, that they might be encountering the same too. Once thoughts differ, it makes a big deal.

It's a pity to see people believing in one thing appearing in different camps. Some remain monotheists and others polytheists because of the same uncertainty of whom to worship. I believe that, in the midst of such confusion, one would definitely be tempted to bring in someone who could bring order. And for that, I personally thank God for those who took the courage to come and teach us about some perfect God who owns it all and deserves all the worship of mankind. This, and only this, makes sense. There must be only one who stands above all and who, even amid the sharpest disagreements, can command order and peace and regulate all.

Unfortunately—and this is the most shocking thing to many—this most worthy God was presented to Africans in two different versions. The God of Christianity seemed to be living in one heaven and the one of Islam in another. (I've been talking about these two religions all along because they're the biggest in the world today and they remain the most influential on our continent. Judaism, Buddhism, Hinduism and even ancestral worship are nothing in comparison. Other religions don't seem to be so close and compelling to Africans like Christianity and Islam. We always refer to Christianity and Islam when talking about religions in Africa).

If these gods are different, as they're portrayed by their followers, then there is not much difference between them and our primitive ones. There again, the "freedom to choose" is called back: one feels he must be left alone and be given some time to figure out which of the two gods is worth following. The choice here may still be based on the performance of the two gods because definitely one should be better than the other. Only a few people would go for a bad god because no one enjoys badness for its sake, and the majority would join the good god because often goodness is appreciated mostly for its sake: goodness is good.

So, whoever teaches about these gods (whether a Christian or a Muslim) must always remember that people—potential adherents—need to be given time to make their own free choice before they join any god because it's a matter of figuring out beforehand which of the two is good and which one is bad. That's why forcing anyone to join your god is not good, and it shouldn't even be any god's responsibility to do so. We live like machines, with our "free wills" serving as fuel that makes us run. We're given "free wills" to make choices.

Finally, whenever people talk about these two religions they only mean eternity. All their talk, however complicated it may seem, simply means that there are only two options offered in eternity: heaven and hell. Both are attained by one's choices before he dies, and this includes even the choice for the type of god he decides to join. So, everyone's choices now affect his destiny in a great deal. Whatever one chooses to do or whichever way he chooses to behave every minute or second determines whether he'll be a heavenly or a hellish creature in eternity. Therefore any choice, especially the choice between gods, should not be taken as a game for children.

Now people are very intelligent creatures; they are aware of all this. Some who have never had any such idea learned it from others. Then, I guess, the person who learns something about these gods would be ready to accept any of them (provided he's good) because otherwise hell awaits him. And whatever ideas we have about hell or whichever fanciful beliefs we may have about it, we never forget that hell is just hell. It has nothing likable: there's nothing good about hell. And that's how far so many people have come along.

For that reason, I think it's far better to be a bad person joining a good god than being a good person joining a bad god. Because when you join a good god your badness would likely disappear as you are surrounded by an overwhelming goodness. But when you join a bad god, no matter how good you might be, the badness of your god would choke any attempt to be good. And both your goodness and the badness of your god will be broken into pieces some day in future. The good god will ultimately triumph. And that would be the end of all stories about religions, thus letting eternity to unfold—and everything else after that is unknown to all of us.

That's why anyone who knows about this is so afraid of making a quick choice. Forcing him to join any god would therefore be a merciless act. This is a matter of life and death, and if that is what it is about choosing these gods, one would always want to do it alone. When he goes to hell, it would be for his own recklessness or obstinacy; if he goes to heaven, it would be because of his "ability" or the grace he gets for having made good choices.

Persuasion may be a good method to employ in order to draw people to our gods. Forcing someone with swords, guns and all kinds of intimidations to join our gods is, I believe beyond any doubt, a heinous act that could bring anyone into the pits of hell. Furthermore, persuasion leaves room for choice, and to a greater extent, it accommodates atheists and agnostics but coercion doesn't.

Forcing people into our religions might be profitable and worthwhile only if the aim of our religions was limited either to filling up mosques and churches or to get people to behave in a certain way. But if it's far beyond that—if it's attaining eternity where only heaven and hell are the only two options—then "free will" is the thing that must be encouraged to work. Even our conscience, deep in us, condemns us for forcing anybody to follow our decisions in such a serious matter as this: death or life, joy or sorrow. I believe some people will become friendlier, feel happier, and laugh each time they meet in heaven with the person who aroused their conscience by persuading them to join his good god. Other people will live in a continual hatred in hell with those who forced them to join a god who was just a bad god in the end. So, don't force anybody when it comes to making a choice between gods, just persuade him to join, thus allowing him to make his own good or bad choice—to go wrong or right on his own, so to speak.

We are suppressing our development for nothing. We refuse to cooperate for nothing. Our "Holy Wars" in the name of our gods are only making them wonder how confused we have become. They're only laughing at us their followers because we've deviated alarmingly from their great mission. Let's stop such kinds of wars on our continent. Everyone is free to respond, to proceed his own way or to join any other god. And that's what free will means. Our only task, if we would engage into the persuasion business at all, could be to tell our fellows about the goodness and the loving kindness of our gods. And also to advise everyone to look back when he hears the call: to listen to their voice. After reminding them of that call, we just have to walk away so to allow them make up their minds to either go back, proceed on their way, or join another god.

If we happen to win them through persuasion we would do exactly what is expected of us: guide people to a free and voluntary union with God. This, I believe, is the intended original plan: to be freely united to God through voluntary love. If love is not built upon the foundation of a voluntary union with someone, it's simply hypocrisy—and where there's hypocrisy, the word "love" should never be mentioned. Repulsion is the only result we can ever get whenever we try to bring love and hypocrisy together. And if it's so, why should we bring them together? Apparently God doesn't want a bunch of hypocrites; he wants to gather men and women who would be united with him voluntarily.

Let's stop killing each other. Let's work hard for our development. Let's not wage wars on behalf of such gods who don't expect to see everyone back some day or celebrating with them. They're well aware that some people would spend their eternity in hell for their stubbornness while others would live in heaven for their obedience. Therefore, trying to draw everyone to their side might be a task doomed to an eternal failure.

But people must be reminded or persuaded often because the soul that will freely accept the call is unknown—and the time of the day, or the month of the year, or the year of someone's lifespan when this will happen is unpredictable. I guess if there's any endless job on Earth it is this one because as long as there are stubborn chaps among us (I mean those who ignore gods' calls), then persuasion business will always target them. And I must tell you what nobody should ever plan to do: if there's anyone planning to stop this business, as some individuals and regimes have earnestly tried sometimes back, he must think as well how to plan to fail.

But we must let the gods deal with their people's souls. Since they're the makers of those souls, they may also know how to convince them and draw all those rebellious and stubborn souls closer to themselves. They know the right formulas to employ to win them and above all, they know what substance they're made of and how they can delicately handle them. But if you want to see the opposite happening, I would suggest you some strategy: "Just tell your gods to change the whole system. They must take away the "free will" faculty from everyone and cancel the judgment day." That could work. But if it isn't possible (and we all know how impossible it is), then don't kill your fellow who chooses to remain stiff-necked to your gods' call.

This is perhaps how things will go on for the rest of the human history, and even the reason for the judgment day, so to speak. Don't substitute your gods by already choosing some punishments for your fellows who refuse to join them. Doing that would be anticipating the steps. Maybe, from gods' plans, they don't even deserve such punishments for their wrongs. Maybe there's a specific punishment tailored for every wrong. You wouldn't know because that's not part of your business. If your concern is to see those reckless and obstinate chaps suffering double punishment, don't take it as your responsibility. The right way to get that done would be to tell your gods to catch them on the judgment day because this time it will be a face-to-face encounter: the spiritual, infinite, divine being one side and the natural, finite, human being on the other; and punish them as strictly as possible for their rebellion. Since they're the ones against whom all this rebellious anti-god propaganda was made, they would know the right kind of punishment to inflict on all the rebels.

Let's develop. Let's not waste our time, energy and money in that kind of war either in thought or action. It's useless to both our gods and us. We must rather invest our time, energy, and resources in working toward the development of our continent. Let's focus on Africa's development, not on useless wars.

# Chapter Nine

# The Quest to Build an AIDS-Free Society

AIDS has become a big threat to our continent's development. The universal fact is that today's youth are tomorrow's leaders. Unfortunately, Africa is losing a large number of its youth through HIV/AIDS. This reminds me of my first year at university, when one of my lecturers was teaching on social contemporary issues and the topic was HIV and AIDS. Somewhere during her lecture she said that she was only teaching useless youth when referring to us. It was so comic, the way she put it. Everyone, including myself, laughed loudly at what we thought was a strong joke. Not the reaction she was expecting! Suddenly her face changed and she exclaimed: "I'm serious, I'm not joking."

This was because the result from the blood that was voluntarily donated by some students for test proved the majority was infected. She was worried about the young and precious lives we were about to blow and spoil, that's why she called us useless youth who would probably not serve our countries after we graduate. To me, it didn't matter that much at that time, but now it's crystal clear that she was arousing some sense of responsibility in us. The responsibility of reversing HIV/AIDS is in our own hands. In other words, each youth could be held responsible for our present state. The task is ours to choose: either to die of HIV/AIDS by being pigheaded even in the midst of advice or avoiding it by applying some prevention measures.

Statistically, Africa is the most affected continent and its youth is the most infected. We need to do something to eradicate this disease so to save the youth—our potential leaders. Without them, development is impossible. That's why HIV/AIDS is discussed in this book.

I'm going to mention its cause then I'll suggest its "cure." I know it's not easy to get people's attention when you talk about HIV/AIDS "cure;" that's why I'd simply say that I believe in its prevention, which is feasible and possible if only there'll be a psychological shift in Africans' mindset. And, that's where our hope lies.

I strongly believe the rise of HIV/AIDS infections lies in ignoring abstinence. The only principles upon which to base our lives today should be, as C.S Lewis put it, "complete faithfulness or else abstinence." Here, for some reasons, I'll not deal with "faithfulness," but every married man or woman must remain faithful. Now this is so difficult and so contrary to our instincts because, I'm afraid, our sexual instincts have gone dreadfully wrong. Sex is nice and very enjoyable, but abstaining from it is far better, especially now.

In my life I've noticed that all the things we see as nice are also the most dangerous. Sex is one that has brought us all the most complicated diseases. Food is another, because obesity and all its vices are basically caused by it. Money is also among them. Almost a third of all the most awful evils we are facing in the world today come from the ambitious desire to get more of it. But power is the worst, I think. This confirms the old saying, "Too much of everything is bad." On that saying could be added, "and every misuse is costly." We must learn not to acutely like things the way we do sometimes, they can easily cause our peril.

One easy way to help us discover how wrong our sexual instincts have gone—or how sex is being misused in our society—would be looking at the increasing number of HIV infections. How many cases of venereal diseases are reported to hospitals on a regular basis, and the increasing number of unwanted pregnancies among our teenagers?

I'm compelled to once again borrow from C.S. Lewis: Is there more abstinence in our society than before? There is no such evidence. Contraceptives have made sexual indulgence far less costly within marriage and far safer outside it than ever before. Public opinion is less hostile to illicit unions and even to perversion than it has been in Pagan times . . .

Perversions of sex are numerous, hard to cure, and frightful. We have been told a solid lie that sexual desire is in the same state as any of our other natural desires and that if only we abandon the silly old idea of hushing it up, everything in the garden will be lovely. The moment you look at the facts, and away from any propaganda, you see that it is not. They tell us that sex has become a mess because it was hushed up. But for the last twenty years it has not been. It has been chattered about all day long yet it is still in a terrible mess. If hushing up had been the cause of trouble, ventilation would have set it right. But it has not.

Modern people are always saying that sex is nothing to be ashamed of, and they may mean a couple of things. Perhaps they think there is nothing to be ashamed of in the fact that the human race reproduces itself in a certain way, not in the fact that it gives pleasure. If they mean that they are right. But if they mean that the state into which the sexual instinct has now gotten is nothing to be ashamed of, then they are wrong. There is nothing to be ashamed of in enjoying food, there would be everything to be embarrassed about if half the world made food the main interest of their lives and spent their time looking at pictures of food, dribbling and smacking their lips.

We are surrounded by propaganda in favor of promiscuousness. Some people want to keep our sexual instinct inflamed in order to make money out of us. In the first place, our warped nature—the devils who tempt us, combined with contemporary propaganda for lust—make us feel that the desires we resist are so natural, healthy, and reasonable, that it is almost perverse and abnormal to resist them. Poster after poster, film after film, novel after novel, associate the idea of sexual indulgence with the idea of health, normality, youth, frankness, and good humor.

This association is a lie. Like all powerful lies, it is based on a truth—the truth, acknowledged above, that sex in itself (apart from the excesses and obsessions that have grown around it) is normal and healthy. Surrendering to all our desires obviously leads to impotence, disease, jealousies, lies, concealment, and everything else that is the reverse of health, good humor, and frankness. For any happiness, quite a lot of restraint is necessary; so the claim made by every desire, when it is strong, to be healthy and reasonable, counts for nothing. One man does this on religious principles, another on hygienic principles, another on social principles. Every sane and civilized man must have some set of principles by which he chooses to reject some of his desires and to permit others. Any natural desire will have to be controlled anyway, unless you are going to ruin your whole life.

It is the misuse of sex that has quickly spread HIV/AIDS and other STDs, and has caused the number of unwanted pregnancies to grow among our youth. Giving in to every sexual feeling has brought us all this mess. We just have to completely abstain from unprotected sex if we want to fight this disease or decrease the number of teenage mothers at all. And for the past few years this has been bugging most of our governments.

HIV prevention, on the other hand, lies in saying "yes to abstinence." We have ABC as principles preventing HIV/AIDS. A: Abstinence. B: Be faithful. C: Condoms. Here I'd insist on "abstinence" for a reason I'll explain later. At the beginning of this chapter I said I won't deal with "faithfulness," but I also advised every married person to remain faithful to his/her partner. For me, only "abstinence" remains the powerful weapon to supply to the youth if we want to reverse HIV/AIDS. One possible question here would be why only "abstinence" and not "condoms," too? Maybe my own perception of condoms would not be so convincing to many. For that reason, I will use what was uttered by a certain head of state. One African leader is quoted to have said, "It seems that condoms are not doing their job." He was the president of one of the countries that invested a lot in fighting HIV/AIDS and where condoms reached even a poor farmer in some remote areas of his country. In his country, condoms were distributed and made available to almost everyone. After few years, he delivered such a controversial speech complaining that the campaign was seemingly "unsuccessful" because the rate of infections kept on rising. He must have noticed that condoms didn't do much to diminish HIV infections. He noticed the "fallibility" of condoms, so to speak. Perhaps his observation was that "the more condoms were distributed, the more people got infected." Maybe this is exaggerated, but the truth must be something closer to that.

I'm not saying that condoms are not effective at all, but I'm inclined to think that they seem to be ineffective in so many African states. The increasing number of HIV infections and unwanted pregnancies in our society shows that condoms are either not sufficient to prevent AIDS or else, they are some magic portions that disappear from our pockets right before the intercourse.

But if they're trusted to be effective tools for AIDS prevention, then there must be something wrong either with our culture or our mindset. Well, I also know that it is quite difficult to get people use condoms effectively in a culture where it is believed that a sweet tastes sweet out of its wrapper. Yes, how would you get a people whose reaction toward condoms is that "a banana cannot be eaten with its peel" use them effectively? But, when talking about sex, bananas and sweets are the most useless analogies to bring in. They are only going to leave us hopeless and miserable in the end. It is also not easy to get people's minds away from sex in a culture where almost everybody believes that "everyone else does or should do it."

First of all, it is not my intention to discourage the distribution of condoms. I encourage those distributors. They must not sit and wait until some imaginary day in the future when our mindset would shift so we would use condoms effectively. The day and time this shift would occur are really unknown. And I will tell you how I think it would work. The psychological shift we're expecting is not like some evolution myth, where all the chimpanzees reached a certain stage of smartness and at once all changed into what we are today and all the previous species disappeared altogether. It's neither like some students in a given grade who are promoted to the next together. What I mean is that the psychological shift will not happen to all of us at once; like when it's winter, everybody will get cold. I believe it'll be a random experience. It'll start happening to some first, then to others, and so on. More like sunshine on a partly-cloudy day, or like the independence of our countries: though every country was entitled to independence, they didn't get it all at once. That's why the campaign for condoms must continue, even in the present time. I wish this shift could happen soon, even this time before I finish typing this sentence.

Secondly, "everyone does it" (or what could be called peer pressure) is, in so many cases, a great spoiler. I know most of us enjoy following the crowd. Unfortunately those following the crowd usually get lost in it. And thirdly, one should not obey everything his feelings suggest. The most ironic fact about feelings is that they are never permanent. Feelings come and go, so why should one pin up all his life on them? Therefore, resisting them—not giving in when they drive us crazy—would be the best practice because they'll definitely go. That's abstinence in practice.

I said a moment ago that condoms are not effectively used in many African countries. This is based on my friends' and my own experience. I would use a condom only few times with a new partner, but if that relationship lasts for a little longer than two weeks, I usually thought my new partner would be faithful to me by then. Diagnosing with my own eyes—based upon looking at her external appearance (a good-looking body)—I would quickly conclude she must be healthy. It's only now that the old French adage that appearance is always misleading makes sense to me. I hardly thought it would contain some bit of truth in it in front of a beautiful girl. This is another kind of opium. It is either drunkenness or addiction.

Now I guess some of you are laughing at how my friends and I were so naïve. For my continent's sake, I should apologize for such a dim-witted naiveté but if we can all be honest, our stories would be similar. That's what most of us do with condoms here in Africa. Today I know my status is safe and secured as result of opting for the first principle: abstinence. I know beyond any doubt now that my life could be endangered if I solely depended on condoms. Don't think that I'm blaming anyone for using condoms. I'm not against them. If there's anyone amongst us who uses them effectively and promises to continually use them so, he is wise. But if one just theoretically believes in their effectiveness and cannot practically use them properly, he's slowly endangering his own life and that of his partner(s). My advice to such people is that they should either use condoms effectively or abstain completely from sex.

I didn't comment on the entire ABC approach in detail, but emphasized more on "abstinence" simply because I believe in its efficiency. But in every other respect, I believe in the whole approach and would love to see it ranged as it is now: in the three first letters of our alphabet (ABC), that is the order of importance, I suppose. The danger I foresee is that of trying to inverse it: CBA. That is the order in which we tend to put them when we're campaigning. We tend to put more emphasis on condoms ("C"). We tell people they're free to go for sex, to gratify their sexual feelings whenever they want to provided that they "condomize." Unfortunately, this has proven to be a failure so far. The increasing infection rates of venereal diseases and unwanted pregnancies in our society prove it. This shows that most of us fail to use condoms effectively. "Be Faithful to your partner" (or "B") is advice given to unmarried (single) fellows. This recommendation appears to be failing due to the fact that our culture seems to hold to the mentality of "tasting every meat on the butcher stands." "Be faithful to your partner" makes more sense to married people or to those who have some life commitment, as it seems to be a complement to the conjugal promises made to each other in court, at church or before families, friends and other witnesses. The principle of abstinence ("A") is pushed back to the third position because the majority of us think it's impossible to abstain from sex before they even try it out. But the possibility or impossibility of something is tested by a serious attempt.

Therefore one is "allowed" to go for sex, but with a condom or one partner only. He is told to abstain only if he feels he's strong enough to resist the feeling or if he's ready to starve himself sexually. So, all the people we refer to as being "old-fashioned," clinging to some archaic beliefs (and I'm not sure if I can be spared from this), should stay without sexual partners. In that way, being carefree or perhaps outgoing when it comes to love and sex is considered as proof of civilization or at least some kind of advancement. And I'm always left to wonder in which sense such a problematic indulgence could become advancement. That's not how we can reverse this dreadful disease. For most of us in Africa today, freedom means switching from one sexual partner to the next. And in this way the virus gets more hostages.

I think this freedom from any guidance outside ourselves is the most deceiving ally to us in Africa; else we must either be misusing it or misunderstanding it altogether. Though I deeply dislike imposing rules or drawing bottom lines for other human beings, when I think how sex is stirring brains on our continent, I'm tempted to review my belief. Maybe people should be dictated what to do or how to behave when it comes to sex. Perhaps our governments should consider that. However, there's no neutral ground on this issue: It's either you let people off or you squeeze them. I'm afraid of being dubbed otherwise if I go deep on this subject, and for that reason I'd rather leave it here.

The right order of these principles, when campaigning for HIV/AIDS, should start with a strong emphasis on abstinence, followed by faithfulness to one another. The third option, if one can't abstain (which I believe everyone can and should, especially with the present state of things on our continent), or be faithful (which I also believe is not impossible), he can do whatever pleases him provided he uses condoms. Condoms must therefore be the last resort if the two first principles fail. We must promote and apply ABC, not CBA. That's how we can help our countries and our beloved continent in general. Instead of forcing our countries to spend more on antiretroviral medications for the huge number of our fellow infected folks, we can just apply the ABC approach and get our way out. Then our money would go for development instead of purchasing those expensive tablets. Let's be zealous to apply ABC. We can make it, guys!

To conclude this section, I would like to say the following: it is unwise to overlook the doctor's prescription. ABC stands as our three recommendations from doctors. Doctors' recommendations, when well observed, prolong one's life. Our case is similar to a diabetic who is advised to eliminate sweet foods from his diet, or an athlete whom the doctor advises to stop practicing because of an injury he suffered. Unless he takes it as a joke, he would never reduce such advice even by an inch. Even if it means to sacrifice his entire career or his enjoyment, he would go for it if he were serious. And for our own case we have to be serious indeed.

Stopping some people from eating sweets stuff may be akin to telling them to forget about food altogether. Likewise, urging an athlete to stop doing his sport is like telling him to forget about big money. It's not an easy experience, but for the sake of his life, one has to make some tough decisions and keep them. Such are decisions we need to make and keep now.

On our continent, HIV/AIDS is taken as a story for kids or a big joke. That's why so many people are still reluctant to apply the principles of prevention. Maybe this is because it has been discussed for decades now. People are getting so used to those campaigns that they no longer amount to anything to them. As a result, they go on doing whatever they want without caring about the consequences that might follow their piggish indulgence. The most shocking fact is that even when they're agonizing in their beds, they still cling to some utopia that some evil spirit or some witch in their neighbourhood must be responsible for their suffering.

AIDS is real, friends. It's not a manmade story or a shrewd strategy invested by some moralists or religious fanatics to stop us from enjoying sex. It's a real disease killing millions of people every year, especially on our continent. I'm afraid of being taken as a storyteller too. But I don't care about anyone's beliefs now; I have the same message to all of us: AIDS is real, and nowadays everyone is expected to take some serious precautions.

# Chapter Ten

# Let's Help Them Out!

There's another issue I didn't want to leave out. It concerns people I sympathize with and who I see being marginalized, in a way. These people are being treated like devils of hell almost everywhere. They have never been taken like full-fledged people, with minds and all. Often they're considered as semi-humans, perhaps due to their traumatized minds. People think they can only perform badly even if they try their level best. It's difficult for them to be easily accommodated or integrated into local communities. They always go unnoticed even if they try hard to fight for their rights.

The most shocking thing is, the more they fight for their rights, the more people stop listening to them, perhaps because of trauma. Those who look after them and even their hosts are quickly annoyed by their complaints which they quickly dismiss or reduce to "nonsense." Whatever they plan, think of, say or suggest is questioned and referred to "trauma" first before it could be taken into consideration after a bundle of corrections, rebukes and checkups. Whatever they touch is automatically seen as dirty, whatever they wear is unclean, whoever gets closer to them is likely to contract a deadly disease. That's how they are unfairly stereotyped!

The people I'm talking about are refugees and asylum seekers. They are the ones treated this way. But in my view, if there are any people who need assistance, refugees and asylum seekers must be the first. They're forced to move out. Like an African Proverb that says: "It's only the grass that suffers the damage where two elephants are fighting." These people are really innocent ordinary citizens.

They are busy with their crop-farming, school activities, typing their essays and their book chapters as I'm doing now, selling in markets and on the streets, fishing in the rivers, dams and lakes, playing by moonlight, telling fairy tales around their evening fires, going to and fro, and performing their daily chores when everything starts. I mean when those greedy and selfish guys amongst their fellow countrymen sign contracts to take up guns for money, power or "change," these ordinary men are not invited. They are unaware of the whole story.

It's only some time later, after the war breaks out, that they are given some fallacious promises in the name of liberation and change. They don't even welcome the change in question. Even if they could accept such change, I guess they wouldn't expect any machine gun to be involved in the process. Now we must get this clear: it is one thing to be a citizen of a country and yet another to engage into an act as outrageous as killing his countrymen for money or power. But most of us forget this when we accuse refugees and asylum seekers for their countries' unrests. We assume that all of them are, in one or another way, architects of any problem arising in their nations. That's a completely wrong approach.

Some of these people are busy performing their daily chores when suddenly someone or some group get them out of their activities. In a minute they have to run from schools and offices only to find nobody home or everybody moist in their own blood. They have to leave their goods in the shops and on market stands to get support and relief from their neighbors. I guess the majority of them don't want to get in their neighbours' territory because they need nothing like support or comfort before the situation gets terribly worse. Some of them are satisfied with their crop-farming, primitive life, which make them needless of their neighbors' support. Their daily businesses help them live without bothering much about getting any glimpse of what's going on next door. They live peacefully. Isn't self-satisfaction synonymous with peace, anyway?

The idea of getting out of their countries comes in as soon as their houses are put on fire, their sons are killed or forced to join the army, their wives and daughters are gang-raped, and their possessions are looted by some greedy compatriots. It is only after all this that they think of seeking support and relief from their neighbors. As a result, all of them are found squeezed in a corner of their neighbours' territory. At this time, their biggest desire is to see their neighbors sympathizing and identifying with them in such time of need. Their urgent need is to get some attention, care, and comfort from their neighbors.

Unfortunately, all they get back from their neighbors is a "we-don't-want-you-here" attitude. Suddenly they get all kinds of evil names. They're accused of bringing in all sorts of contagious diseases after only few days in their neighbors' territory. Well, how can someone escape cholera in a concentration camp? Their children die in their hands. They're told there's no sufficient medication, meaning: "There's only enough for us," or "You are too dirty to be admitted in our hospital wards."

Where should such people live? At least some place is chosen for them. And it is often a remote place—a place where life has never been easy for anyone, including citizens. Some are put in the middle of the jungle, where they must cut down many trees before they can secure a space to pitch their tents. Others are sent to live in some dry places where water is to be transported from kilometres; they're confined to some indescribable places.

I'm not against concentration camps. If refugees are put in these camps in order to facilitate census for their identification and assist them easily while they're all in one place rather than scattered around, it's a good strategy. But if they are to be kept in one place so they would not spread diseases, I think it's not good. It's worse than genocide. It's like building a town uniquely for those suffering from AIDS. It's like saying to your fellow brother, "Go home and die, leave us alone."

The right strategy to employ if we want to help those infected with HIV is to allow them to live with us. We must not isolate them. And only our support, affection, and empathy can help them live a little longer. Here, some might be tempted to say, "I don't have to isolate or abandon my siblings or my fellow countrymen; the other guys can go to hell." And that would always bring us back to the same evil we are trying to combat: "selfishness." It might be a patriotic statement, but it's also a discriminatory one. The adage, "a friend in need is a friend indeed" is also true with a neighbor. We must always strive to play a fair game with anyone we meet on our way, including our neighbors.

The question that I may possibly be asked here is why should one allow all the trouble of making space for everybody (including his neighbors) in his mind? Well, if that is a trouble I don't know, but I know about something that we can't easily get rid of and which we didn't invent: our longing for a just and fair world. We do not simply talk or sing about it because we love the slogan, but because we find in ourselves something compelling us to behave so. Secondly, each one of us should try to answer the following question before he does anything: "What would be my reaction if someone else plays rough with me?" I think the reply to this question refutes any of our yearning to send our neighbors to hell, because that would not be fair at all.

Often our decision to play rough on our neighbors is motivated by thinking that we will never bump into them in our entire lives. We think nothing could work in their favor to make us need them, too. No one knows what the future holds for us. The world we live in is full of surprises. (But we must stop wishing bad luck to each other. That, too, is unfair). We must therefore be mindful that whatever we do in the present time has future implications.

In soccer terms, for example, we could say that your team may have to play a second leg away with their team some day. And this time, it will be on their home field. How would you like to see that game? Using the terms of this version, we could say that your children might come across your neighbors' children in their court some day. What type of game would you expect to see: a fair game, or a rough one? Barring a miracle, if that game happens to be played at all, with "the-game-must-end-in-a-draw" syndrome in Africa today, your children would be in trouble. They could go through hell because your neighbors' children would use this opportunity to get an equalizer. Whatever that may cost them; I know they would be looking for a draw. We're such a rancorous race, remember. We do not easily let go of anything.

And I know as well as you do that that would never be the end of the game. It would go on and on. And the more it would be played, the rougher it would get. Remember the consequences of a draw game I discussed in a previous chapter. Revenge never comes to an end; it is the bloodiest game one could ever play. Try to imagine a world where everybody is just animated by resentment. That's how it would look like: hell on earth. And by the way we treat refugees and asylum seekers, one is left to wonder if we are not closer to that at all.

Besides, refugees are not as stupid as most of us think. Even though some of them are traumatized (and we know why), they have heads, arms, and legs just like everybody else. Their only disadvantage is that they find themselves very destitute in their neighbors' countries. They have no money and lack every other basic commodity. The truth is that they can do better than some of us. They are very clever. Another fact is that they are not carriers of any deadly diseases. Those diseases attack them as soon as they get into those concentration camps where they're forced to live. If anyone doubts that and wants to get an unbiased answer, he must simply look back where they came from to find out whether people have been dying of those terrible diseases or not. If the answer is yes, then they should be isolated or even deported back as soon as they step into their neighbors' borders. But if not, integrating them into the local communities could be an effective therapy to cure all the diseases and abnormalities associated with them. And here the choice lies in the hands of their hosts. I mean the choice to allow them enter the house. It is their neighbors' choice to either allow them get into any room or let them use only one corner of the kitchen and punish any trespassers.

But how do we expect people from many cities, villages, and hamlets now confined in one camp to be free of cholera or other dangerous diseases? The terror (to both visitors and even hosts) starts in those concentration camps.

My suggestion on this matter is that we must help, love, and support each other; especially in times of trouble. My wish is for us to build a continent—or even a world—where nobody would be displaced because of violence.

International humanitarian bodies take care of refugees and asylum seekers, but we must not leave it all up to them. How could we depend solely on foreigners to take care of our neighbors? They do a great deal of work, but I think neighbors could empathetically assist and care more than some strangers because they're aware of what's going on next door. They witness the madness. They should at least give more support than some faraway foreigners, or at least selflessly work hand in hand with those humanitarian organizations instead of leaving everything in their hands. If one brings money, jobs, capability, space (land) and all the likes in, everything would quickly collapse. It's better to ignore that first and offer what you can. .We must help refugees out; they're our brothers in the real sense of the word. But if we don't want to consider that or are unable to meet some of their needs, we should at least give them a warm welcome. We must sympathize with them as our neighbors. Let's practice and promote the politics of good neighborliness.

In my summary, I would like to say that "Einstein was a refugee" poster displayed in several places could convey two positive messages. One is that refugees are capable of doing better work than people think, and some are geniuses. Do not despise nor undermine them. Another message is that being a refugee is not something to be ashamed of. Do not let anyone discourage or look down on you because you're a refugee.

The first message goes outwardly, while the second is more introspective. But, in every other respect, I think it would be better if every refugee learns to master his inner man.

To me the first message is sent by people fighting for their self-worth; it tells outsiders that they're clever like everybody else and that, given the opportunity, they can perform wonders. Therefore, no one should ever despise them. The second assertion goes inwardly. It's like a consolation from one's friends, but it's also like a tender pat from a loving and caring mother to her hurting child. Here, refugees are told to accept their status, for it brings no harm on them and it doesn't affect their minds or anything else they have. At least this can give them some hope.

Before I talk about the message "Einstein was a refugee," I would like to start by saying that no one should take this poster as a mere advertisement intended to appease or to do some good for refugees. It is true that Einstein was indeed a refugee. The poster's message is that refugees are not people from some strange world: they are citizens of a certain country who did and can still achieve great things everywhere they go, when given the opportunity. They're good thinkers and strong people. They're refugees simply because they fled their countries and are now looking for help, comfort, shelter, protection, support, care, and rescue—which they had never thought to solicit before—from someone else. But that has changed nothing about them.

So whenever we see refugees flooding into our countries, we must know that they mean no harm; they're only after the shades of our houses. We have no choice as to whether to welcome them or not; they have already crossed over their borders and now they're in ours. They can't return to their homelands because everything they left behind is on fire. The only thing that survived is them. They need everything we have to survive, and more than anything else they need our sympathy. So, let's try to give it all to them. We must try our best not to hold back anything that could help them survive.

Albert Einstein once was a refugee, but now is among the most intelligent and renowned men of our world. His achievements are known everywhere, not because he was once a refugee but because his refugee status didn't diminish his potential. His achievements talk more than the status he once had. I wish I knew the autobiographies of many African leaders who once were refugees, too. I also wish I had some permission to mention their names in this book, but luckily enough I know most of them and I believe most of you know them better than I do. If presidents, members of cabinets, permanent secretaries, CEOs, governors, soldiers, and others in key positions in many African governments today were refugees, then there's no doubt that any other refugee in our countries today stand the chance to become an influential leader in his country someday.

Whoever comes as a refugee needs our support and deserves it. I also know that some of them are what I call "fake refugees," for they take advantage of the situation to hide behind "real refugees." They cross other countries' borders illegally, taking advantage of free services. We should just help anyone on the continent who comes as a refugee, no matter what. But if we can easily detect fake refugees and discover genuine ones it would be a wise thing to do. We must go ahead and do it. What I'm afraid of when I say we shouldn't discriminate against them is that if one starts doubting some, he may end up doubting them all—and then the real refugees could suffer. They must be sustained, and here is where I put my whole emphasis. Helping them is more like helping the whole country—I mean the entire nation, from leaders to subordinates. No wonder why some countries have got such strong relationships; perhaps it's because of some fair play games during such times of trouble some time back. Some good games were played long back, now what we see is their outcomes: prizes—the handing over of some medals, so to speak. At least in this case, one can clearly see some good side of fair play in times of trouble.

Well, I've been advocating and propagating for unselfishness. One ought to be unselfish for so many good reasons. Selflessness quickly draws us closer to others. We tend to stick closer to unselfish friends. Now if you ask me what the use of being unselfish is, I might not be able to give you a straight answer except for something that would bring us back to where we started. It won't get us any further if someone keeps on asking me why one should be unselfish, because I'll simply tell him that we all like people of such character. Then if he asks me why should one bother about what benefits others if his self-gratification and pleasure are more important to him, I would tell him that people don't care about the standard you set for yourself if it hurts them. At this point, I guess he might complain, "It's not fair when people hate me for my own standard." And when he says that he'd be caught, because "fair" is a word without meaning if only one side benefits. Fairness means what makes both you and me happy at once. If you expect other people to be fair about your lifestyle, you ought to be unselfish. And at this level we are back to square one. It's a vicious circle.

Unselfishness and fairness echo from the bottom of our hearts. Something inside each one of us compels us to behave kindly. It's then a personal issue either to ignore or obey it. We feel and hear from deep within us that we ought to be unselfish and fair regardless of our own fancies. And I know am not bringing in any new philosophy; it's one that everyone knows about and complains of when he doesn't see it function in another person.

I would like to summarize this chapter in some practical words: "If there's only one tree in the desert, all the birds' nests will be made on it." Here I want to talk specifically about southern African countries. These countries, like South Africa and Namibia, are full of foreigners from all over. Why do all the people come to these countries? Perhaps it's because of their modern facilities and various opportunities. Remember in my first chapter I said the dream of an African is to live in a paradise some day. I can't imagine anybody who would endure hunger when he hears that his neighbors are throwing food in the bin. Who would not look for a better shelter if his was leaking? Who would not solicit a ride if he were tired of walking? Who would not look for a monthly remuneration if he were fed up with forced volunteerism? Who would not look for a job if he feels he were well able to work?

This litany of questions can be endless. The above questions explain why southern African countries are overcrowded by people from all over our continent. Southern Africa seems to be the only tree that is still surviving in this desert of Africa, and there's no way it can avoid all sorts of nests. Every bird (big or small, tidy or untidy) would be enticed to come and find shelter from it; and every kind of nest (big or small, dirty or clean) would be made on it. Now southern Africans must not be frustrated by the presence of foreigners in their countries. Now that they know they're the only tree that is surviving in the entire desert, they should be proud of their state. I mean they should be proud of their achievements and be willing to take the challenge of leading all those other crumbling nations There. I mean to show them how development could be achieved. They must always know that we're in the process of getting "There" from "Here," and accommodating each other is one of the ways that will get us all "There" pretty quickly.

Our experience shows that the weak cleave to the strong for protection. By "strong" I mean order, security, the rule of law, respect of gender, good governance and public management—in a word, democracy. Fellow southern Africans should keep foreigners within their borders, which could help the continent reverse the great challenge of massive one-way clandestine migration to the West. They must always remember that if their house is the only beautiful house in the vicinity and the rest is only a bunch of huts, they are likely to receive visitors of all kinds and from everywhere, arriving at any time of the day with various needs. When that happens—as it is happening today—and those who have nice houses want to stop it, they can teach others the secret of getting and maintaining a beautiful house. As soon as they learn that, those intelligent learners among their neighbors may automatically start building their own houses and probably stop crowding southern Africa.

Of course, some may adopt and apply it as fast as possible, while others may be slow to implement the knowledge. Some are innovators, some are early adopters, others adopt later on, and yet others lag. The difference between them is their time of adoption, but they all have one thing in common: The spray of the new idea or innovation reaches them all—no matter how far they may be standing. Instructors must be patient with them. They must continue helping them to come out of such extreme dependency. In more practical words, I'm talking about helping them to get peace and to be economically free in some way. And I'm happy this is happening now. Many southern African leaders have been fully involved in the process of reconciliation and peace building in central Africa and other wounded regions of the continent. If they carry on doing that with the overwhelming desire of developing Africa, they could be doing exactly what would quickly get all of us "There" from "Here."

We visitors must be grateful for the welcome we receive from our hosts, and then we must always remember that we are still liable to any "host-guest bond." This means that we must continually behave decently in order to leave the house as clean and tidy as it was before our arrival. We must not scratch the painting, destroy the ceiling, break the windowpanes, mess up on the floor, or misuse anything in our reach.

We must live in their house always reminding ourselves of our status as only visitors. During our stay (and this is where our intelligence is required) we must listen carefully to our hosts' counsel and seek to apply what they are telling us to do, even before we move out. This could be our training session. We must be ready to take their advice in order for us to build our own beautiful house later and achieve autonomy. We must get rid of pride and put on humility. We must open our minds and listen. This is what we should always remember: we got attracted to their house because it was in good order. And if this is true, then it qualifies them as lecturers of development for the rest of us.

Finally, here is where our wisdom is called back: when we succeed to build our own houses, we must remain kind to them. No matter how modern, beautiful, strong, or clean our new houses may be compared to theirs, we must always remember that they helped us reach the level we reached. So, we must endlessly apply the politics of good neighborliness: to play fairly. We must keep in mind that it's all about brothers or sisters (or at least neighbors) living in the same yard, wanting to keep their milieu as attractive as possible to meet the requirements of entering the competition with other yards.

# Chapter Eleven

# Zulu's Wishful Thinking

This chapter is based on a dialogue I regularly had with one of my friends at university. The reader must be informed that the choice of the name Zulu is intentional. I first was attracted by Zulu's name because it's an African name. You cannot mention it twice anywhere before someone remembers its origin. However, this name was chosen not only to describe a tribe in South Africa or a descendant of that tribe, but it is the proper name of an individual, a Zambian artist in a small town of Mbala and a university colleague with whom I spent four years of my undergraduate studies at the University of Namibia. He was very inspiring and encouraging to me during all the time we spent together. So many times we shared ideas that we thought could help to develop the continent in one or another way. And it's those words I've reproduced here. Nevertheless, they are not some strange stuff; they are rather day-to-day topics or wishes of the continent. They sweep across all generations and age groups.

The wish for Africa to be one huge country dates many decades back in the era of independence. Leaders such as Kwame Nkrumah, Patrice Lumumba, Julius Nyerere, Jomo Kenyata, and others constantly showed their longing for Africa to be one right after many countries achieved independence. They were foreseeing African unity not only politically but also in every other aspect. The Organization of African Unity (OAU) was basically created for this aim, and its successor, the African Union (AU), has the same aim.

Most recently, at their meeting in Libya, African leaders seemingly couldn't agree to make Africa one huge country in practice. I believe we all see in the same way and share almost the same feeling despite some small disagreements arising amongst ourselves around this issue.

Zulu's wishful thinking on this topic is not a lone one. It is the belief that Africa will never improve if we do not unite all our resources and skills. We look weak and therefore prone to failure because we are so fragmented. And often outsiders take advantage of such division to manipulate us like toys. But if we united the little strength we have, we could probably be able to stand against outside challenges and pave our way to a brighter future. One of the benefits of such unity would be the freedom to move about and run our businesses wherever we want; this would likelier allow us to get employed in other states with less difficulty. This would strengthen our economies and advance our development. In fact, the union of many states is pivotal to any regional development. Unity is indeed strength. We have seen it in the case of United States of America. I guess that's why the U.S. was a bit indignant toward the European Union when it was formed. And now it wouldn't be surprising if the two unions show the same attitude to our own unity, because they know what such unity is capable of achieving. But if, against all the odds, we ultimately manage to unite, we would get "There" pretty quickly.

When Africa becomes one huge single country, an Egyptian would easily purchase his goods as far as Cape Town and sell them in Cairo at an affordable price because he wouldn't spend much on custom fees. Imagine the excitement of an Egyptian in a remote village buying a South African-made product at nearly the same price as a Cape Townian.

I guess some of us would argue that free movement would give way to an uncontrollable massive one-way migration, as in the case of South Africa and other southern African countries that are full of foreigners. But Zulu believes that one-way migration movement is caused by tight control and strict conditions we put on people who wish to travel around.

When Africa becomes one and if a Senegalese was allowed to work in South Africa, he won't have any problem with visiting Senegal every weekend. He could even run some business in his state after he has gathered sufficient resources to start such business. But even if he gathers wealth in some faraway state and still remembers how much he has to spend on visas and custom fees alone before he gets to Senegal, he'd cancel the trip. As a result, he'd be forced to prolong his stay in that country and live there—even clandestinely or with some forged documents. And that's the cause of one-way migration movement in our continent today.

Or if a South African farmer could be allowed to get land in DRC without many hassles, he would be able to employ many jobless Congolese youngsters flooding Kinshasa streets. And how would such youth mind to enter Zambia, South Africa, or Namibia or any other country through irregular channels if they receive almost the same wages a Namibian farm worker receives in their state? Or how would people starve to death in Ethiopia or DRC if our own farmers were producing enough food that would easily be exported to other states with less custom fees or at a free cost?

It is beyond doubt that regional organizations on our continent, such as SADC or CEDEAO, are being devised for the same aim of trying to ease some of our national or regional problems. Isn't that we wish to live in a place where our goods are not charged any custom fee, where we would use the same currency, enjoy cheap electricity from our neighboring countries, get water for irrigation from other countries' rivers, and cross several borders without bothering much about visas? Zulu believes that is exactly the idea behind all our regional organizations. Other continents have seen the benefit of that and have implemented it.

At this level, our challenge is that some of our countries seemingly believe or think that they cannot survive without the money generated from visas and custom charges from foreign traders. Maybe it is still difficult or too early for Africans to implement it. Or perhaps it's difficult to think of some corporate good in a world where individualism marks the order of every single day. I wonder how European countries managed to overcome some of these barriers in our time. I also wish we could learn some of their secret power, but I'm not sure if we should take Europe as our point of reference. We must just do it our own way. But taking Europe's strategy as reference is not sinful. Anyway, that's one of our wishful thinking.

Zulu also thinks that corruption of all kinds is yet another barrier to our development. Unless we reverse the situation, we won't progress any further toward development. And so our journey would become more difficult. Africa cannot get developed if corruption is not dealt with accordingly. Most of us, especially those in leadership positions, seem to be corrupt to the core. We find all forms of corruption in Africa. Bribery, for instance, is out of control. It's been exercised in different ways and has different names according to regions or milieus. In some countries, no service can be rendered to anybody without a payoff. It's being made official, and, in fact, seems to have become a right. No official can offer any service without expecting some extra money. Likewise, anybody for whom the service is rendered tends to feel like it's robbery or unrivalled ungratefulness to walk away without adding something on the normal charges of the service he receives. It's in this way we have damaged everything in our countries.

People from outside our continent never understand why they should buy lunch for government clerks in our Home Affairs Ministries and other public agencies. A Tanzanian gospel singer expresses his frustration over this in a song. He narrates how he was asked for bribery in some strange terms. In the song he says how he could not understand the terms he was told to make him forcibly bribe an attendant in a public office. He was told to pay "something small." He didn't understand what that meant, but the term was quickly changed to "tea" before it was finally changed into "cool drink" following his failure to understand even the second term.

In DRC, for example, bribery is called "madesu ya bana," literally meaning "beans for kids." And sometimes people are asked some silly questions such as, "Do I eat papers?" to mean that you brought papers (documents) and I attended to you but papers are not edible. That's only a few examples of different names attributed to bribery that I could recall. This is how awfully spoiled our continent has become. And most of this is happening in public services.

I know this has to do with someone's attitude first, because if someone's nature is corrupt to the core, it's pretty hard to help him change. In order to offer any help in this regard, we need to work with the psychological part of individuals first. But when you delve into this issue, you'll find out that it takes more of social stance than psychological. How do you expect a police officer with a family under her care to arrest an irregular man who offers her more than her meager wages? How do you expect any public servant not to beg or even force someone to pay him for a service rendered while he goes several months without salary? Who would take care of their families and other daily assignments of life in a world where only money seems to be the only answer to everything? Therefore, it is evident that though one could have psychological features upon which to act rationally, he would be forced to do otherwise because of all the expenses under his care that his salary fails to cover. Naturally, men are among the best survivalists in the world. They would always find alternatives whenever some other avenues are shuttered. That's one of their survival strategies in times of deficiency. Maybe, apart from seeking psychological therapy, our governments should first seek to increase our public servants' social packages and wages if we want to combat bribery or any other type of corruption.

In most of our countries, only those who have money are quickly attended to, especially in public offices. Sometimes this "tea" or "cool drink" or "madesu ya bana" is twice the normal charge for a particular service. I once heard that in some of our countries the normal tariff is doubled whenever it's a white man who is requesting a service from a black attendant. Maybe bribery is also a racial thing. Maybe!

Yet in other countries immigration officers hunt for foreign nationals to cunningly draw money from them. Likewise, some of these foreigners bribe immigration officers in advance so they can turn a blind eye on their fake documents or any other irregularities. This scenario is really out of hand at the moment. The danger of condoning corruption is manifested when the country's safety and security are at stake. Some of our nations were and are easily being lost to foreigners because of money. When we all become coin collectors, who would care what the briber does in the country? Unfortunately, in such countries every business is permissible. No game is forbidden in the territory of coin collectors. "Do whatever you want as long as you drop something in my bank account" seems to be the rule of every single day in all our states. And, sadly, there's no better way to describe Africa than that.

Heads of states or concerned ministers do not appoint managing directors of mining or oil companies or any other highly generating service who cannot guarantee them a return. Their appointment is based on how much they're willing to drop into their bosses' accounts on a regular basis—how to keep their bosses on track, so to speak.

The education system of some of our countries is in complete shambles due to corruption. And how do we remain on the competitive edge if we learn nothing valuable in our schools? Education is the basis of all advancement, yet most of our countries have only a shadow of education going on in their schools: no new curriculum, no qualified teachers, no classrooms, no laboratories, no libraries, no desks or tables, no chalks, no books, no papers, nothing essentially educative. Now what is left to be called education in all this?

What is our diamond and oil doing for our continent, let alone our countries? When those we call leaders are driving the most expensive and quasi-unaffordable German and Italian makes, living in fancy houses in countries where the population is dying of hunger on a daily basis; where children whose poor parents are forced to pay teachers do not attend school; where the rate of death rises considerably due to lack of medicine and appropriate tools in hospitals and clinics; where public servants and even those in uniform go years without remuneration—what would you call all that?

Furthermore, we remark unspeakable human deficiency when it comes to elections in Africa. Some politicians think they have the right to twist the results of elections as long as they can command those in uniform or maneuver other governing bodies in the country. This has been repeatedly happening around the continent, and often voters' complaints are either overlooked or silenced brutally. We must always aspire for peace, transparency, fairness, freedom, and credibility of elections, but aspiration alone does not stand as bottom line. Our bottom line should always be the maintenance of such peace and transparency and their maintenance during the few hours or days of the exercise. Any flaw or fraud during such exercise should be indicted. To our potential leaders, what to retain is that if elections do not mean the end of a term—thus determining who should continue or come into the office—then the whole exercise is meaningless, and therefore do not seek for anyone's participation. Hence, millions of dollars spent in the entire process is an unspeakable waste. And it would be true foolishness to make such exorbitant expenditures for simple formalities.

Yet the message is that if voters really matter, then their decision should matter, too. It should not be taken as some formality, though that is indeed how politicians treat our votes: *simple formalities*. It is useless to invite people to participate in such an exercise if their votes don't count or have any impact ultimately. Stealing elections is morally defective. It undermines African values to the core. We profess these values all around the world because we believe they are creditable.

You cannot persuade men and women old enough to be your grandparents to spend several hours in long queues under the scorching African sun and twist their free, wise and precious choice at last. We have lost every sense of morality we used to hold so dearly, and indeed which used to describe who we are.

Sadly, some heads of state, members of the cabinet, parliamentarians, and other senior government officials think the country's business starts and ends with them. In truth, it starts and ends with ordinary citizens, and that is what our leaders should learn. After all, we are all ordinary citizens before we climb any ladder of leadership. It is quite shocking to see most of our leaders maintain two such camps at once in those offices. One camp is for those who have successfully crossed the dividing line into a new camp that permits them to patronize others; the other is of those below the line, left to be beggars solely depending on the first group. Parliamentarians are no longer people's envoys to advocate for the need for potable water, health centers, transportation and communication, electricity, and other basic needs in the parliament. They become too complacent once seated in those parliament houses. Once they have achieved their dreams, they have crossed the dividing line—and everyone else is left to strive their own way to make it to the top.

On the other hand, our politicians have taken us captive because of our own attitude. We allow them to cheat on us so easily. No wonder why we have become so cheap to them. We have been hearing the same stories in all their propaganda but we have never lived any differently afterward. And, deplorably, we have never questioned this or challenged them for this. In fact, we have never held them accountable for their talk after they win elections. They promise to respond to our primary needs—water and electricity, new schools and cost-free basic education, employment, improved road infrastructure, good salaries—but often nothing materializes. They come up with the same stories again when campaigning for another term and we attend their rallies in numbers and excitingly applaud the same fallacious promises before ultimately voting for them. One wonders what makes us so forgetful.

It's time that we learn to take our leaders on their words. It is also time that our leaders learn to walk their talk. We are sick and tired of the status quo in Africa and would like to move from where we have been stagnant for years. And when we move we shall be able to change the last statement of the chorus of the AU anthem. It will no longer be "Let us make Africa a tree of life;" instead it will be "Let us make Africa a paradise."

Besides, how could we achieve development in a continent gone mad like ours? We watch our fellow brothers die of hunger while we throw food away, we watch them struggle with the most devastating poverty while, in some of our prosperous states, we sit on the surplus and keep millions in our private or even public bank accounts. We watch them being exploited while we have the power and ability to defend them. We watch them go through many awful experiences in life that, at first impression, would have even a visitor from another planet think that we're selfish brats. Yet we seem to respond to that with a "Who cares?" attitude.

The most shocking dilemma, though is the fact that we watch and even support wars elsewhere on the continent—killing millions of innocent people each year—simply to get money in return. Ironically, we claim that the wave of democracy has reached us. Yet one is left to conjecture what we mean by that. Millions of dollars are expended or even borrowed from other continents to "ensure" peace, stability, and the respect of human rights. Yet in the meantime lots of money is spent to support some of the worst violators of human rights who we know would ultimately shutter all our peace prospects.

Nothing is as breathtaking as seeing how silent we ordinary citizens are vis-à-vis some extreme disparities in our own law practices. Our justice has gone completely awry. All our laws are flawed; all countries without exception are guilty, yet no pressure is exerted to challenge such unjust laws. All our laws are tainted with gender, racial, religious, political, philosophical, and especially social differences. The law that sentences an armed robber, a drug dealer, or a livestock thief to prison for many years is the same law that deliberately or shrewdly spares those in high ranks in our states for unspeakable mismanagement of our public treasures. Even in Muslim countries where Sharia laws are very tight, you can easily notice how they are pockmarked with holes of injustice. A woman caught in adultery is stoned to death under Sharia law, but you hardly hear about the fate of the man. And this list of injustice is exhaustive. Are we to sit and watch? That's only if it doesn't bother us at all.

Looking at our continent today and when considering our practices, is it not an appalling confusion to distribute mosquito nets to fight malaria—while in the meantime we allow violators of human rights to force children, their mothers, and pregnant women to leave their homes and look for shelter in mosquito-infested riverbeds simply to get ore and diamond in return? What is it if not confusion that makes us spend millions in educating children in the endeavor to fight illiteracy on our continent while we allow rebels to force the same children we have been pretending to love so dearly into the army in front of our own eyes? This is the highest form of corruption.

All the evils mentioned above are what Zulu and I used to view as impediment to our continent's development. We should seek to eliminate all of them by all means if we want to achieve development. Development is hard to achieve in a world where such things prevail. Let's develop our continent.

www.ingramcontent.com/pod-product-compliance
Lightning Source LLC
Chambersburg PA
CBHW051437280526
45785CB00003B/1320